LIVING IN LEGACY

ovarian cancer from cell to soul

a memoir

ALEXIA MONACO

Cathy, for you...

Living in Legacy is a select collection of personal experiences, reflections and published references, independently written and printed exclusively for altruistic purposes. It is not intended as a physical or emotional guide, nor as a tribute or critique. With consideration and respect for involved individuals and institutions, many personal and clinical details have been omitted. Subjects have been consolidated and general references are extensive, I sincerely hope to have done them all justice in accuracy and acknowledgement.

Living in Legacy's list price has been minimized to maximize accessibility, any proceeds will be donated to the Ovarian Cancer Research Alliance.

To my army of skilled and compassionate clinicians,
who rescued my body and mind…

To my extraordinary family, friends and acquaintances,
who lovingly restored my soul…

I am eternally blessed and grateful.

Living in Legacy is inspired by my oncologist,
who encouraged me to consider my legacy, and to live my life.

"Be as a bird perched on a frail branch that she feels bending beneath her; still, she sings away all the same, knowing she has wings."

Victor Hugo

THE DIATRIBE

"Read widely of others' experiences in thought and action–stretch to others even though it hurts and strains and would be more comfortable to snuggle back in the comforting cotton-wool of blissful ignorance!"

Sylvia Plath

Mirroring the size and shape of an almond, the ovary is nothing more than a small ovoid structure and nothing less than the paired heart of the female reproductive system. A baby girl is delivered with all the eggs that she will ever have. Over the course of half a century, from birth to menopause, one to two million potentially viable ovum will dwindle down to one to two thousand infertile remnants that will lay waste. In addition to their hoarded cache, the ovaries busy themselves producing reproductive hormones that orchestrate the complexities of monthly menstrual cycles over the course of nearly four decades. If we dare to peek behind the curtain of what defines sex, we will find them ruling a woman's anatomy and wielding the ultimate power to give or take life.

In *The Ultimate Guide to Ovarian Cancer*, Benedict B. Benigno, M.D. describes ovarian cancer as "an avaricious tumor and its domain is nothing less than the entire abdominal cavity. It can extend from the deepest part of the pelvis up to the diaphragm, to the right and left of the colon, and everything in between. It can appear after only a few weeks of the mildest symptoms, and by then it has already declared open season on the body of a woman. It is fiendishly difficult to treat and unrelenting in its destructive ambition. It is a modern-day scourge casting a narrow and selective net, forever changing the lives of its victims. It is one of the most difficult diseases to diagnose and the most lethal of all gynecologic malignancies."

1

Ovarian cancer may be one of the best kept secrets in the medical world. Statistics are bleak and longstanding, with no clear cause and the field grossly lacking in general awareness. Despite great advances in treatment, oncologists must violate the primary tenet of their code of conduct and, with the best of intent, first do harm. Grim mortality rates are excused by a lack of proactive diagnostic testing and the cost of a conversation has been discounted. Evaluations have yet to be standardized, and women are charged with identifying and reporting the semi-silent symptoms of advancing ovarian cancer.

The disease whispers, and we must save ourselves.

THE ONSET

"We are most deeply asleep at the switch when we fancy we control any switches at all."

Annie Dillard

With a bevy of repentant sins under my belt, I will soon reach for reason and it all started with Eve. From the Garden of Eden, to antiquated libido references in the 1800s, to more intellectual, less maternal roles in modern times, Mother Nature's revenge falls punishingly on the ambitious childless woman for not following a traditionally prescribed path. She is most vicious with her own kind, and I had it coming.

*   *   *

I've known privilege and ease, recklessness and responsibility. Born into gifted circumstances, I was reared by personally and professionally accomplished parents. As an only child in an adult world, I was nurtured with equally loving measures of structure and freedom. With inclusive global perspectives amid a culturally rich environment, I was taught the values of character, resolve and self-reliance. Favored with genetics, inspiring examples and vast resources, my conditions are seemingly ideal.

Never without inspiration and opportunity, my path has been largely self-wrought and fluid. Ambitious, impatient and independent since my formative years, my sense of self has only intensified with age and experience. I am determined, am not easily intimidated and rarely do I cower. As a collaborative leader by nature and productive perfectionist, control is something I relinquish only when my confidence is high or it pleases me to do so. Equally strategic and creative, I am accustomed to options, choices, prospects, escape.

My husband and I have realized the future we had envisioned

building when we imperfectly leapt into a life together. Too enamored with each other and our dreams to not take a sledge hammer to our prior marriages, I also abandoned my home, career, friends, family and community to enter an unknown fray. We grossly underestimated the collateral damage, the eggshells we would tread on, the landmines we would avoid, the price we would pay.

*   *   *

In lieu of the nimble limbs of children, my wanton hips bore designer clothing and the imprint of countless forgettable hands. Against all odds, I avoided the wrong man at the right time, though I did once envision legitimate motherhood. I even went so far as to undergo fertility treatments in my first marriage to compensate for biological inadequacies that were not mine, to no avail and unknowingly ticking off one more correlating risk factor.

Seriously entertaining the challenge of an unrealized aspiration, I had pressed the issue early on with my current husband. Eighteen years my senior with three nearly grown children, it was too late for us, too complicated.

*   *   *

Never wicked in my role, I naively presumed that my stepchildren would suffice to fill any resulting void, undervaluing the influence of a privileged upbringing and the acrimony of a mother scorned. Later, armed with the knowledge that childbearing reduces risk, I will wonder if I might have spared myself had I taken an alternate path. If my husband's extensive acts of servitude are retribution for difficulties bonding with the children borne of a loveless and likeless marriage, and not ours.

From temporary and likely baseless musings, I redirect to my reality. I am fulfilled and at peace with what I do and don't have. Not having borne children of our own ultimately yielded our precious liberty. Of my many regrets, this is not one.

Though guarded and cautious from the wounds of a rough start, with an open mind and heart, I hope for softer threads to be woven into the delicately-knit fabric of our disjointed brood. I am deeply committed to and appreciative of the family that flanks me, both by blood and, even more so, by beloved choice.

*   *   *

As impetuous as our union may have seemed, our marriage has stood the test of time. Our lives are purposeful, we have worked for and attained an idyllic state, extraordinary in both love and life. We have established a meaningful and inclusive foundation with our family, friends and community. My career in international business management has been as challenging as it is rewarding. Following my husband's retirement and his sensitivity to his father's early and untimely death, we have been making up for our missing memories and spending more time realizing our shared passion to explore the world. We are at our best together and growing in consideration for ourselves, others and our environment.

My world is perfectly intact, vibrant and rosy. I fall asleep to a kiss and wish for sweet dreams and wake to a kiss and promise of a good morning. Neanderthals and savants, my husband and I have our own language and communicate with sounds and chickadee *fee-bee* bird calls. We know each other by heart. By taste, scent, sight, sound and touch. We are nearly one, separated only by my sixth sense.

Presuming myself exempt from downfall, I am blind, deaf and dumb.

IGNORANCE IS BLISS

November 2019

"We are pathetically eager to believe that, if human affairs are managed right, nothing unpleasant need befall anyone."

Max Hastings

November marks the introduction to my year of reckoning. Despite being well versed in routine wellness matters and health care, I am oblivious to the links between the arbitrary and easily discountable issues that I have been recently experiencing and the deadliest gynecological cancer of them all. Like a bad apple, my skin reveals no blemish but I am rotten to the core.

*   *   *

Memorable now and discountable then, I live with the harsh clarity of hindsight. During the last year I have noticed occasional abdominal fullness, nausea and bladder pressure, though never in an alarming or persistent manner. After a piggish order at an atmospheric historic tavern in Virginia, I was instantly nauseated as plates were delivered and unable to dine…yet enjoyed every other meal on the trip. I canceled dinner parties on more than one occasion and miserably powered through one without eating…yet hosted other innumerable parties enthusiastically. My mother expressed concern, which I, of remarkably strong and stable stock, dismissed with false assurance. Minor, random and rare, these issues resolved themselves without further consideration.

Always and still slender, I have altered my wardrobe, favoring full, loose tops and avoiding cutting waistbands. Adjusting tight jeans to rise above my waist when sitting has become a habit that my husband comments on. My stable form appears to be in flux, though I haven't gained weight or changed clothing size.

On only a few occasions do I remember being distinctly aware of generally feeling unwell, oddly tired, lacking energy, disinterested and worn out. My many voracious and insatiable appetites are slightly quelled, deadening. Perhaps showing my age, I am forty-six years old and dismiss the occurrences as developing dietary sensitivities to dairy and gluten, or changes in metabolism. I am disappointed, embarrassed, and silent.

*   *   *

I have not consciously connected a single dot, it is only my vanity that spurs action. In one of countless shower epiphanies, in the weeks prior to my annual wellness exam, a moment's disgust with the slight distension in my once taut lower belly leads me to decide that I will file a formal complaint.

*   *   *

Following my regretfully slight scheduling delay, in mid-November I meet with my primary care physician, intent on mentioning feelings of abdominal fullness during our appointment. When I casually do so as we are wrapping up our visit, she discounts nothing.

To our mutual surprise, she notes that I have actually lost weight. When she taps on my abdomen and percussion reveals a dull tone to her trained ear, I sense her concern and experience my first moment of breathless stillness. Quickly recovering confidence and control, in the first of many failed self-diagnostic attempts, I presume that my bladder is distended and suggest that I go to the restroom and that she re-examine me. She declines and orders an abdominal ultrasound instead.

Aware and attentive, I ask what she senses, what she suspects. Confirming that something is amiss, she is on the hunt to find the culprit to my complaints, possibly a benign tumor. Sheathed in the ignorance of model physical and emotional wellness and a nearly immaculate medical record, I am easily reassured. Immediately astute, she is the first in line to save my life.

*   *   *

My husband accompanies me to appointments. Though we are generally joined at the hip, I do not invite him into exams and my tension levels rise during our ride home. I am self-conscious, as if this abnormality is a shameful pregnancy or filthy sexually transmitted disease, to be hidden away and dealt with quietly and swiftly. I am intentionally dismissive when I tell him that radiology has been ordered and hesitate to mention the possibility of a tumor, to address a complaint that I have never voiced.

*   *   *

My first act of preservation is controlling exposure and intake. I prioritize my privacy and limit distractions. I swear off research rabbit holes and stay grounded exclusively in my medical team's information and advice. Soon to come unhinged, with just a few keystrokes I could have uncovered the truth. Lost my will, succumbed to the statistics.

*   *   *

At the first inkling of a crisis, I draw open the curtain to my medical modesty. My husband will play an active role in all aspects of my care. He will charter me to every appointment and delve into every detail. There is nothing he will not sacrifice for my wellbeing.

Against my husband's wishes, I elect to disclose nothing to my loved ones until we know more. My intentions to not inconvenience or distress my family, friends and colleagues are well considered. Most concerningly, I know that my parents will be upset and feel betrayed. Our relationship is close, open, and supportive. I am wholly confident in a judgment that I will later come to deeply regret.

*   *   *

One week later, I lay on a table in a dark room having the prescribed abdominal ultrasound. I watch the technician take multiple images and measurements, study her impassive face, knowing that she is trained to not reveal what she can surely interpret. Following a worrying conference with the radiologist (whose report will suggest we consider carcinoma), she returns to release me. I am miserable and finally able to empty my intentionally distended bladder.

*   *   *

I am home alone hours later when my doctor calls to introduce me to the sizeable mass residing in my abdomen. She has sought and found a 17cm x 16cm x 11cm complex cystic structure. Comfortably settled, it is a rude and invasive guest, fingering its way throughout my abdomen, overtaking and oppressing my organs with wild abandon.

My doctor expresses surprise that I have not been experiencing significant digestive issues (though I will later learn from my nurse that my age and general fitness enabled me to better mask and tolerate symptoms). I have kept calm and carried on. Built for childbearing, my mind is accepting and lacks the neurological warning signals to refute a foreign presence. My body has been accommodating, making way deep within the cavity of my womb for the savage tumor consuming my vitality.

*   *   *

We cannot continue to cohabitate, and my doctor provides me with a surgical referral to a gynecologic oncologist. Word association is incredibly powerful in this setting and hearing my doctor's first reference to oncology is startling.

Though cystic masses are generally benign, when I ask about exploratory screening, I am advised that a biopsy will not be conducted…to ensure containment, should the mass be cancerous. When I ask if the surgery will be a minimally invasive laparoscopic procedure, I am advised that it will be a maximally invasive open procedure…the mass is too large to be excised through a tiny hole. When I ask about timing, I am advised that it will be in short order…the mass is infringing on my vital organs.

Still in a state of ignorant bliss, I am entirely unaware that my body's whispers over the past year are classic telltale signs of advanced ovarian cancer.

*   *   *

From positions of power and authority, I quickly assess and gain control, strategize, and take deft action. Approaching challenges as expeditiously as I would in a business meeting, I am an assertive facilitator, identifying all the components, purposes and players, clearly in charge when making appointments and filling out forms.

I contact the oncologist's office and am given the first available appointment on December 4th. Orders are placed for a CA125 tumor marker blood test and an abdominal CT scan. Results will be discussed during our visit. Orchestrating to our mutual best interests, my husband and I intend to meet with my parents that afternoon, with clarity and a plan. While recognizing the circumstances as unforeseen, I am totally oblivious to how my existence is swiftly transferring from my control to providers and medical facilities that are unknown to me.

Never having experienced a health crisis, I inexpertly busy myself and quell panic by developing a tidy and efficient plan of action, to be flawlessly worked into our existing schedules. I investigate likely surgery timelines and recovery periods. At best, I can expect a two-week recovery and schedule surgery in early December or January, without interfering with our family's upcoming holiday or travel plans.

*   *   *

Possibly psychosomatic, I become hyperaware of a foreign presence in my body. My lower right back aches and I can now see and feel more significant abdominal distention, though no one else would be the wiser.

My husband avoids touching my belly. With restrained contact, I feel ashamed and unattractive, grossly flawed.

I take turns cursing it as an entity unto itself and companionably referring to myself as *we*. Along with bouts of nervous giddy laughter that I term *tumor humor*, I face waves of panic. I reflect on feelings of discomfort over the last year and changes in behavior, my awareness and recall growing.

*   *   *

A CA125 is the first of hundreds of blood draws that I will have in the coming months. I don't make eye contact with the syringe and dread and despise the invasive poke, every single time. I will always abhor needles. So much so that my abhorrent anticipation yields far greater cumulative angst than needles ever will on their own, yet I will fail to be desensitized.

An abdominal CT the week of Thanksgiving promises insight. I drink the tasteless oral contrast fluid in the outpatient testing lobby. We are eventually taken back to a radiology department lounge, where I anxiously await being prepared for IV contrast as well. Another patient can be heard from behind a privacy curtain, making a fuss and requiring multiple technicians to administer her IV. The dramatic commotion in advance of my own procedure provides perversely inappropriate comic relief. My terrible propensity under pressure to laugh at the most inopportune times has turned into gallows humor. In this setting, it is surely a coping mechanism to displace stress and fear.

11

The technicians are professional and compassionate. My IV is inserted with nary a peep from me. I am advised that I will experience a rush of warmth in my groin when they inject dye during the test, that many patients have the sensation that they are relieving their bladder. When my eyes widen, they promise me that there will be no actual bedwetting!

With my slightly southern etiquette always intact, I maintain clinical cocktail party mode and welcome a polite exchange regarding what symptoms and events preceded my visit. Of all things, I'm bothered by the inorganic contrast mediums and will be sure to purge them from my body with copious amounts of water. What I should be more bothered by is the radiologist's report, which will indicate that findings are worrisome for carcinoma. I receive a heartfelt hug and well wishes as I am leaving. With that telling goodbye, another thread unravels.

*   *   *

When a questionnaire from the oncologist's office arrives in the mail, I promptly complete it. Other than the noted symptoms, I feel stellar and have maintained all activities. Timing is of the essence, yet I do not hear the tick-tock, the beating on the drum...

Returning from one of our daily walks, when climbing the stairs to our fourth-floor condominium unit at a good clip, I note a very mild, though abnormal, shortness of breath. In the moment that I pause on the last stair landing, hesitating to take the next step, I recall that one of the oncologist's questions relates to shortness of breath. Had I not just read that, there is no doubt in my mind that I would not have noticed or given it a second thought. I waver for an instant, considering that I frequently experience an increased heart rate and breathlessness nearing the last leg of the climb. This is different, though barely so. The warning is nearly imperceptible.

Reluctantly, I change my answer from no to an alarmingly lifesaving yes. It's bone chilling to realize how something so minor, so ignorable, so unremarkable, so dismissible, can be so deadly.

*   *   *

In our bubble, we contain the possibilities. In ancient Greece, *kosmos* described an orderly and harmonious universe. Conversely, in *khaos* everything fell endlessly in all directions, with no solidity, no up or down, no earth or sky.

During what may be our last Thanksgiving celebration, I will be the one to take a family photograph, standing at the opposite end of my parent's kitchen island and already removing myself from the picture.

*   *   *

Stress fractures begin to form, yet everything I know and trust in myself has not yet shattered. I have not been betrayed by my body and mind. I am not yet crippled by my real and perceived strengths.

With appreciation and high regard for the professional resources surrounding me, centered in self-reliance, I know nothing of their depth and how they will serve and save me. In fine health, I do not know the staff, services, systems and facilities whose excellence and responsive efficiency I will rely on for my survival.

A giver by nature, I do not know the bounty of close and extended family, friends and acquaintances that will soon gather in force to surround me with their care, assurances, prayers, well wishes, expressions of support, love and admiration.

*   *   *

Secretly, I begin to live on bated breath, suspended and powerless. Under threat, I am frozen, motionless and tense. I vacillate from feeling nothing to a dreadful sense of consuming panic.

During one of our many walks, I am overcome by a rapid heartrate, shallow breathing, tears and intuition. I have a very bad feeling.

*   *   *

Fear is clawing its way into my psyche, though I am still whole enough to harness my emotions. I calm myself with assurances that I am immune, protected, safe.

LIFE VERSUS DEATH

December 2019

"Like all explorers, we are drawn to discover what's waiting out there without knowing yet if we have the courage to face it."

When Things Fall Apart, Pema Chodron

The cancer center sign looms large on the building, it is breathtaking. Despite the intimidating and deeply saddening setting, I am feeling quite well on December 4th when I meet my gynecologic oncologist for the first time. Prepared for a conversation regarding surgery, we unknowingly cross the threshold from the before into the after.

*   *   *

If my oncologist has a complex, it isn't visible to the naked eye, though she will be my god and save me. She connects with me with focus and authenticity, giving me her time freely. Encountering most of her patients for the first time in an emergency, she is quick to establish a rapport and garners immediate trust by facing me directly and with intimacy. Within minutes she lends structure and familiarity to the surgeon/patient relationship, which is so foreign and frightening to me. She calls me her friend, which I know I'm not, though I appreciate the connection. She is building a link that is familiar and nurturing, giving me something known to cling to.

*   *   *

If I wasn't securely perched at the foot of her examination table, my oncologist could easily knock me over with a feather. CT results refute psychosomatic symptoms, I have imagined nothing. My uninvited boarder has made obscene gains and now measures an impressive 20cm x 18cm x 12cm, yielding a staggering 44% increase in volume over the course of one week.

Ill mannered, it is compromising my kidney function, delivering extrinsic compression to my bladder, and must be surgically evicted with haste. (Optimistically, I presume that I will be recovered well in advance of Christmas and our plans for the new year!)

CA125 results are in range and deliver confidence that the tumor is benign. Presenting the worrisome alternative, my oncologist uses the *C* word, citing a 15-20% chance of ovarian cancer. A dirty word, cancer is uncomfortable, unnatural, unbelievable. I apply a stigma to my reproductive abnormalities and the disease, pornographic shame.

*   *   *

Trying to understand the possibilities, I seek answers but cannot pin down the cause of a cancer that has no reason. We discuss general correlations, including not being in the baby-making business and an ironic absence of birth control, as well as potential triggers, like environmental toxins and stress.

Accepting that it's not an actively preventable disease, it's especially torturous to live with the knowledge that I might have spared myself to some degree. Assuming responsibility, had I known the warning signs, I am confident that I would have reacted more promptly in bringing the seemingly insignificant issues I was experiencing to my physician's attention sooner rather than later. Had I only been driven to report at on-set, listened, reacted, advocated. I will own and suffer the woeful consequences of my many dismissals, the veil has been lifted.

*   *   *

When she advises that ovarian cancer is not curable, I face my mortality for the first time. In *Memoir of a Debulked Woman: Enduring Ovarian Cancer,* Susan Gubar lays out a harsh reality– current remedies do not cure the disease. "Instead, they debilitate the person dealing with it until she barely recognizes her mind, spirit, or body as her own. Enduring ovarian cancer mires patients in treatments more patently hideous than the symptoms originally produced by the disease, while ovarian cancer itself endures as it has for centuries, unchecked in any significant way by the new findings of contemporary science."

Doomed, I recognize my ignorance and what it may cost me. In a state of disbelief and detachment, I ask my oncologist if she has read Atul Gawande's *Being Mortal*. She has, and when I question cure versus containment outcomes, she assures me that this is no time to throw in the towel. My age, general physical health and supportive environment are valuable and will position me for success under her care. Yet, omniscient, she encourages me to consider my legacy…

*   *   *

I am scheduled for an exploratory laparotomy, resection of abdominal mass, unilateral oophorectomy, bilateral salpingectomy, possible total abdominal hysterectomy (given my age and pre-menopausal state, she hopes to salvage at least one ovary), possible bilateral salpingo-oophorectomy, possible staging and any other necessary procedures. A general surgeon will be on hand, to assist her as needed.

In lay terms, my abdomen will be surgically opened to examine my abdominal organs and cavity for disease. The identified mass will be removed, along with my yet to be visualized left ovary, both fallopian tubes and, possibly, the whole of my reproductive system beyond my vaginal canal.

To boot, my surgery will take place on the most feared day and date combination in history. Since the early 1300s, it has been associated with misfortune. Be it quirk or coincidence, evidence points to both Friday and the number thirteen being unlucky. Hopefully, no one on my Friday, December 13th surgical team suffers from friggatriskaidekaphobia.

*   *   *

Our meeting seems set to conclude, were it not for my reported shortness of breath and presentation of tachycardia. Sparing us the alarm of her clinical concerns, I am led into additional STAT testing. Her efficient staff swiftly take control and administer an EKG and I am dispatched to the nearby hospital for a chest CT.

In the waiting room, I observe other patients. Some are being held post-procedure for results prior to release and I all-knowingly tell my husband that their conditions are serious.

Confident going into the scan, when being walked back to the lobby I am told to wait, I will be summoned to a private conference room to receive my oncologist's call with results. Stunned, I realize that I may not be going home, though it's too unconscionable to believe. I'm one of them! How can that be?

*   *   *

When we are called back, I am conscious of every step towards the room, towards the small table in the back left corner, towards the telephone, towards the answer. I'm nervous when I pick up the handset. The instant I hear her voice, I know that something is terribly wrong. Her tone has changed. We have only just met, had one conversation, and yet I recognize her swift transition from confidence to concern.

Generally a difficult diagnosis, due to a wide variety of nonspecific clinical signs and symptoms, she advises of extensive acute bilateral pulmonary embolisms (PE) and instructs me to proceed immediately to the emergency department (ED).

Facing the terror of abrupt death, with quick shallow breaths and tears, I am wholly unnerved by the gravity of my condition. Reeling as we exit the room, I wonder when and where my husband might have unexpectedly been widowed by his seemingly healthy wife.

*   *   *

Entirely ambulatory, when objecting to wheelchair assistance I am informed of hospital protocol, unaware of my code blue status. In my first experience as an invalid, I am ashamed to be pushed through a crowded ED waiting area, and of all things, to be wheeled past our local homeless veteran. I drop my head and look away from his matching chair, hoping that he doesn't recognize us.

Under immediate intensive care, I transition to the role of compliant patient. In minutes, I am reduced from competent independence to following instructions to change into hospital attire and asking permission to keep my own socks on.

My husband will manage nearly all communications with our family and friends while I isolate myself in the unspeakable. My plans have come completely undone.

*   *   *

In my infinite wisdom and perfectly controlled world, I spared my loved ones unnecessary worry. My intention to meet with my parents in the afternoon following my appointment in a position to provide them with a clear view to the situation and solution failed. Instead of protecting them, I will burden my husband and traumatize them with a conversation that I could never have anticipated.

I don't know how my husband will find the words to explain the circumstances, and I imagine their bewilderment. My parents both spent their careers in healthcare and are experienced and aware. How will they absorb being told that their daughter is facing a medical emergency, being instructed to come to the hospital? Now past their cocktail hour and well into a fine

19

dinner, I imagine their inability to understand or process the conversation, their clueless drive to the hospital, careening out of control. Protesting only weakly, I fear that we will endanger them, ruin their night when nothing will change should we wait until the clear light of the next morning. My husband leaves me no choice in the matter and steps away only once, to make an unimaginable phone call.

*   *   *

I wonder what befell our happy little family. Before blessed, protected and insulated in our collective knowledge, now cursed. In recent years, both of my exceptionally physically and mentally fit parents faced and conquered their own health crises, with lessons in rising to the occasion. The youngest of us all by far, I have unnaturally derailed our well lived and planned lives, instantaneously becoming a physical and emotional burden to my husband and to my parents. What I gave them and what I took from them will always weigh on me.

Incapacitated and tethered to monitors and IV heparin, I watch them all walk towards me. Led by my husband, my mother is a comforting force, and I see my father cry at my expense for the second time in my life. Caught completely off guard with my first emergency hospital admission, my father jokingly threatens me, promising bodily harm when I am released and proving that if I suffer from pseudobulbar affect, it is due to a paternal gene dump.

I can only tell them how sorry I am, with a broken voice and in tears.

*   *   *

I am hospitalized for three nights under the care of a hematologist oncologist. The socks that passed ED scrutiny are never-ending cashmere that seem to go halfway to the moon, requiring an aide's assistance to remove and replace with hospital gear.

During the course of my hospitalizations, I will never be without a familiar face and advocate. My stoic husband will spend every night in my room with me, calmly and reassuringly holding sentry. He will sleep on the sofa under the window, too far away to touch. When he briefly hunts and gathers in the cafeteria, or rushes home to shower and change clothes, I will be watched over by my parents. We will navigate our new terrain as a united family.

*   *   *

Around midnight on the night of my admission, seeking the source of the PE, an ultrasound is conducted on my legs. I listen to the murmurs of the scan as the technician runs the wand over my legs repeatedly in silence. Convinced that she is finding multiple blood clots, tears stream into my hair and I look for my husband's eyes in the dark.

The relief I feel hearing that my legs are clear is immediately displaced with panic when I am informed that the PE likely originated from my abdomen. The odds of malignancy have increased to 50%, though surely every professional that I have encountered already anticipates the diagnostic outcome that awaits me.

To protect my lungs and heart from additional blood clots, I will undergo a procedure to install an inferior vena cava filter (IVC). Never having known that such a thing existed, a retrievable umbrella-like wire filtering device is guided from the right jugular vein in my neck to the inferior vena cava in my abdomen. I am now a card carrying IVC member.

*   *   *

My father instructs me to fight, he says I have to. Failure is not an option. While on safari in South Africa, we learned that the animals are not aggressive until they are hungry or under threat. I'm not combative by nature, though I do push back and don't stand down. In peril and emotionally injured, my known faculties are lost to me and I cannot find my way. Contrary to his everlasting encouragement, I can't always do everything. Brokenhearted, I tell him I don't have it in me.

In *The Art of War*, Sun Szu dictates "He will win who knows when to fight and when not to fight. If you know the enemy and know yourself, you need not fear the result of a hundred battles. If you know yourself but not the enemy, for every victory gained you will also suffer a defeat. If you know neither the enemy nor yourself, you will succumb in every battle." I know nothing.

*   *   *

All shades of hell have broken loose. My disintegration knows no bounds when my oncologist visits with additional concerns in CT imaging. She politely asks permission to examine me and gently proceeds, shadows evidenced in one of my breasts will be one of few relieved threats. Abnormalities on my liver will require an MRI and are the only issue for which I will accept responsibility, as I reflect on my gluttonous lifestyle. Liver damage is a single believable outcome in all this madness.

*   *   *

Anticipating no issues tolerating the test, my MRI meltdown may be charted in the hospital's most dramatic patient archives. Step by step, cords to my sanity snap, one by one. Being pushed through narrow corridors, untouched by decorative finishes and littered with empty beds, alarming department signage, creepy rooms. My entanglement in heart monitors and IVs, the compatibility change in my appendages at the hands of two male technicians. Perhaps in consideration for my modesty, they encourage me to replace my web of monitors, charging me with an impossible task. Unable to care for myself and not being taken care of by them, I am coming unhinged, losing my grip on an unimaginable reality. The technicians respond to my request for help and mechanically transition the heart monitors around my left breast. Claustrophobia takes hold when I am strapped to the table, and a panic alarm is placed in my hand. They retreat to the safety of their observation tank to initiate imaging, leaving me alone with my terror. With the first shocking bang that rings through my system, I am physically jolted, frantic, and squeeze the ball to abort the test and escape.

With the final cord cut, I have unraveled. The technicians are cold and uncompassionate. They failed me, and I failed them. Abandoned in the makeshift waiting room awaiting transportation, weeping and chanting insistently, I beg my husband and parents to get me out of there. They have never seen me in such angst, yet pretend to be powerless to help. I stay tethered to my wheelchair, seemingly crippled and restrained against my will. I cannot stop crying.

Why do I stay bound to the chair in self-confinement? Why don't I wheel or walk myself out? Why doesn't my family heed my requests? Would we all be arrested, charged and imprisoned? Our compliance destroys me.

*   *   *

I am finally returned to what has in mere hours become the familiar sanctity of my room, completely unhinged and in an inconsolable state of hysteria. Passionate and willful like my hot-blooded Italian mother, I generally maintain my father's baseline amicable and even temperament. From infancy on, I've never been an indulgent crier. I likely engaged heartily at birth and, rumor has it, at home following a favorite food declaration of artichokes and teasing by my less worldly first grade peers. It takes a tremendous amount of effort to push me to an explosive edge, yet I am crying buckets, possibly literally. I imagine the saline coursing through my IV, rehydrating my depleted fluids, and the possibility that I may actually choke and drown in my own tears.

I ask my family to arrange a private session with my seasoned nurse, who has known and faced cancer. In my heart, I do not believe that I will survive. I believe that I am dying, because I am in fact dying. She responds to my fears by telling me that there is such a thing as a self-fulfilling prophecy. That without hope and trust, I will not have the strength or vision to fight. I am told that if I am to survive, I must convince myself that it is possible and believe that I will.

Rejecting the people closest to me with consideration that I cannot spare, I seek calm and hope in a stranger who has just put my future back into my own inadept hands. Miserable, I will not be consoled. I cruelly tell my parents to leave, that there is nothing they can do for me, to go home.

*   *   *

The MRI order is still open, though I hope to evade it. I negotiate unsuccessfully with my oncologist, she will not concede to my request that she investigate the status of my liver during surgery.

Because I must be lucid enough to follow breathing instructions, mild sedation is not an option. With no confidence that I can tolerate another attempt and no time to work my way towards endurance, I elect for general anesthesia. A ludicrous way to go about a simple non-invasive test, on all counts.

A muscle relaxant so fully paralyzes my body that I cannot breathe unassisted, a ventilator sustains me. When I regain consciousness, amnesia relieves only the momentary distress of the procedure. The results are concerning but not dire and my post-intubation sore throat and raspy voice are reminders of my weak fortitude.

*   *   *

My oncologist knows everything about me, and I will learn more about her. In addition to her remarkable clinical skills, she is an accomplished athlete and an inspiring survivor, whose heart was bigger than her life-threatening cardiovascular condition. She balances career and family as a mother of three and naturally administers care with maternal affection, not hesitating to touch me and to connect warmly with my family. Firm and insistent when I try to evade her path of action, she tells me that I remind her of her adolescent daughter when I resist her. I acquiesce as my spirit breaks. Less defiant and more compliant, I release myself to her, allow her to serve me, accept my fate.

I respect and admire this extraordinary woman. She is intense, honest, and I know she wants me to live. I hold onto that too. I want to be an exception, to be her best patient, to realize success for her. The countless assaults that my body will face at her hands are my only chance for survival.

*   *   *

My oncologists dance a calamitous tango, keeping each of their fields protected and at bay from one another. They work together to carefully navigate the risks of treating the embolisms with anticoagulants while planning a massive abdominal surgery. In an ideal world, following PE and treatments, even minor surgical interventions would be delayed six months. In my world, they have only days to eradicate the mass that is aggressively obstructing and consuming my vital organs.

When I question whether I will survive the surgery, my oncologist delivers a confident yes, though expresses her concerns regarding my ability to endure the recovery. The blood thinners that may spare me PE driven instantaneous cardiac arrest will inhibit my body's ability to coagulate blood post-surgery, in which case I may hemorrhage and bleed to death.

Trust has been defined as choosing to make something important to you vulnerable to the actions of someone else. Though I have no choice, I will learn the true meaning of the word and act on it. My life is in my oncologists' hands, and I believe that they will save me.

*   *   *

On day four, I am prepared for discharge with self-injection instructions of heparin every twelve hours. I falter as the nurse patiently attempts to train me. After much hesitation, I stab myself in the abdomen with the needle only to immediately pull it back out, without having pushed the plunger to inject the medication. I ask with sincerity if I can administer it while looking away, though in my hip for fear of poking the bear residing inside me. Laughter dispels the horror of it all and we conclude that my husband will be the one to administer the injections. He is the kiss of life.

*   *   *

My homecoming is warm and welcoming. My mother ministers extra care with dinner. Looking forward to the nourishment of her divine stewed chicken with mushrooms and vegetables, I set her vintage pot on the stove to heat and go about settling back in. I realize the burner hasn't lit when I return to a kitchen reeking of natural gas. Disaster now looms at every bend.

*   *   *

We adjust and spend our week happily and busily preparing for the holidays, in business-as-usual mode.

During our morning and evening injection routines, our shadows casting on the bathroom wall remind me of the shower scene in *Psycho*. My husband is a caring and attentive administrator, patiently allowing the alcohol to dry prior to inserting the needle and using a slow and steady hand with the plunger to reduce burning and discomfort. Systematic and logical, he strives to identify how to go about it in a better way, but the effects are unexplainable. The injections are nearly painless sometimes and cause me to rant and rave at others. I curse the shots hotly and leave my poor nursing husband in despair at having inadvertently hurt me.

*　　　　　*　　　　　*

On the eve of my surgery, the prescribed preoperative colon purge makes me horrifically ill, and I wonder if that alone won't kill me in the hours before my admission.

A dear friend sends me an image of a cowboy holding steady in the saddle of a wildly bucking horse with a rousing John Wayne quote. "Courage is being scared to death…and saddling up anyway."

*　　　　　*　　　　　*

On Friday, December 13th, slightly superstitious, I am hospitalized for seven nights. According to the book of *Genesis*, God created the universe in the same period.

Administering comfort with consistency when possible, I had requested the same anesthesiologist I had for my MRI. Despite being told that she would be available, I am surprised to be greeted by a different doctor. With my parents touting the critical role and high risk of anesthesia during surgery, I am unsettled by a strange face, though expect him to carefully keep me teetering, unconscious and alive.

Able-bodied in the pre-operative holding area, I reach the crossroads to what will inevitably kill me quickly if left untreated and life saving measures that are both state of the art and barbaric. As Susan Gubar so brutally articulates in *Memoir of a Debulked Woman: Enduring Ovarian Cancer*, "Debulking has earned the nickname MOAS from surgeons: Mother of All Surgeries.

The silent or whispering or screaming but ignored killer has advanced unimpeded. Days after a CT image finally identifies the ailment, immediate measures must be taken that cannot be fully estimated or assessed until a long incision discloses the internal organs on the operating room table. There and then, efforts to stop the cancer's growth require surgeons to get up the gumption to gut a seemingly vital woman, removing many of her internal organs. The hardly noticeable symptoms of cancer pale in comparison to those produced by the surgeons determined to excise it."

I bid my loved ones farewell, already disconnecting from an implausible reality. Entering surgery without knowing what it will ultimately entail, my family will be kept informed of my progress, and I will be the last to know.

*   *   *

Compulsive and neurotic, when the dust has settled, I will torment and comfort myself daydreaming and imagining it all in graphic detail. From the scalpel to the staple, and everything before, during, and after. The sharp steel blade slicing through my skin and muscles, from my sternum to my pubic bone. Perhaps someone sneezed twice, above and going around my bellybutton (that would explain the jags in my scar). I envision the abdominal retractor splaying me open for all to see, while impinging my femoral nerve. The discovery and gutting by my oncologist, who is so slight in stature. Her tiny gentle hands inside my body, removing the enormous mass. The scale of one overwhelming the other, or perhaps the beast of a thing was hoisted out via crane or contraption. My infamous libido rising and vanishing into the thin antiseptic air, as all my feminine bits and pieces are extracted and placed on a tray. I ponder the drama that preceded my splenectomy, the inadvertent laceration and extent of bloodletting. How far they let me venture towards a transfusion and death before deciding that the best course of action was to remove it. In my deafness, I listen for the sounds in the room and dialog. The eerie beeps and hisses of the machines and monitors keeping me unconscious and alive. I strain to hear music playing, singing, humming along or a whistle while they work. Conversations about last night's dinner or this weekend's plans, the suggestion that a priest be called in to deliver last rites. Voices soft and hushed or frantic and urgent. Laughter, banter, gasps of fright and horror. What a fucking mess…

I would welcome a recording of the procedure, to still my active mind, to not be both the center of attention and the only one in the room entirely unaware. Both present and absent then, forever discomfited, I will never know.

*   *   *

My surgical report cites thirteen unlucky pathologies. It includes an endometriosis discovery, exploratory laparotomy, resection of abdominal mass, total abdominal hysterectomy, bilateral salpingo-oophorectomy, appendectomy, inadvertent thrombocytopenia induced splenectomy, bilateral pelvic lymph node dissection, bilateral periaortic lymph node dissection, right hemidiaphragm resection, bilateral perirectal tumor resection and staging, as well as a then unknown femoral nerve injury.

In more appalling elementary terms, I have been slaughtered and butchered. My diseased insides are revealed and excised, including endometrial tissue, a monstrous cancerous tumor, every single internal sex organ (sparing and permanently debilitating only my vagina), my appendix and its digestive support, my spleen and its immune support, lymph nodes in my pelvis and abdomen, a diaphragm tumor and a rectal tumor. An inadvertent impingement on the femoral nerve located in my pelvis and running down my right leg will numb the tissues and paralyze the muscles that enable my ability to walk or rotate without my knee buckling and causing me to collapse.

*   *   *

I wake drug-addled, corseted and tethered to machines that sustain and monitor me. IV fluids and drugs course into my arm, an octopus-like central venous catheter (CVC) protrudes from the jugular vein in the lower right side of my neck, a Foley catheter drains my bladder, and an intermittent pneumatic compression device (IPC) on my calves supports my circulation.

*   *   *

Years ago, it was common practice to avoid revealing and discussing a diagnosis of cancer. Since the end of the progressive "Me Decade" in the late 1970s, physicians routinely discuss cancer diagnosis, treatment options and prognoses with patients, while avoiding imminent death discussions.

In a state of post-operative delirium, I cannot recall the drama of the delivery and can cite facts without an ounce of sense memory. Of all gynecologic malignancies, ovarian cancer is the deadliest in its class. Worse yet, there are types or sub-categories. Rare, aggressive and resistant to chemotherapy, clear cell carcinoma was initially termed mesonephroid. In 1973, my birth year, it was officially defined by the World Health Organization as a histologically distinct type of ovarian cancer.

Any cancer diagnosis must carry a base level of devastation, painting its victims with the same damning brush. Cast in stone, staging is permanent and unmodifiable. No matter how successful treatments may be, no matter how much time passes without recurrence, it may not be exchanged or improved upon. There will be no get out of jail free card for me, I am in it for the long haul. A likely fatal stage IIIB diagnosis has been assigned and received, though I am too comfortably numb and desensitized to react.

*   *   *

Everything is foreign and unbelievable in its entirety, other than my deep scarlet nails, which shimmer alluringly. They are the only thing worthy of a compliment from the visiting staff tasked with my care.

An imprisoned convict is recovering across the hall from me. Multiple police officers monitor his room. While he walks the posh hospital corridors with shackled ankles, I note and continue to report that something is wrong with my right leg. I've lost feeling, movement and control.

A gifted rose quartz facial roller lays on my bedside table, it is exactly what I need and I request it more than I do narcotics. Monitoring the crease that has developed in my brow, my husband smooths away the indication of my pain or distress and will continue to do so by hand through the end of my time.

*   *   *

Even on a restricted diet, I am barely eating. The only thing I am compelled to read during my hospitalization are the artificial ingredients listed on juice and Jell-O cups, which I protest. My parents negotiate meals with me for the first time in my life and my husband pleads with me to take one more bite of scrambled eggs or mashed potatoes.

Like King Tut, I am packed up at night with pillows for support and comfort, tucked in and made safe. I will have no sweet dreams. The oximeter burns my finger and wakes me. The IPC reminds me at minute intervals that I am being protected, and that I am at risk.

*   *   *

My hurt is bearable, as long as I don't move. When I do move, it is agonizing. The smallest adjustment is excruciating in a body linked by thousands of connections to a devastated abdominal core. A morphine drip enables me to self-manage pain, though

31

I am chided for being stingy with it while my husband is strictly reprimanded for pushing my button.

Through bullying, my family ensures that I am well medicated in advance of my epic adventures. Three months ago, my husband and I were carrying on with our grand romance and freely exploring Glacier and Banff National Parks. Now, I am too feeble and broken down to manage the most rudimentary acts.

Escaping the confines of my bed requires the push of a call button for professional assistance. An Olympic ordeal, it seems to take forever and a day for an aide, usually young and male, to help me position myself to the side of the bed for leashing. A yellow gait strap is placed under my arms and around my chest, carefully threaded above, below and through my various appendages. Standing is a herculean chore. Too weak to catch myself when my right knee occasionally buckles, I collapse to be painfully caught by my tether.

*   *   *

With a glimmer of ego still intact, I continue to grasp for a fragment of my robbed dignity. At death's door, the first thing I do when I am finally standing is ensure that my ill-fitting gown is properly arranged and tied.

I am 1,000 years old, and every aided and walker assisted step is a feat. Yet to diagnose my femoral nerve injury, I will work with a physical therapist taking sluggish walks and eventually climbing stairs with much ado and at great risk.

*   *   *

The care I require is unintentionally demeaning and degrading. My traumatized digestive system is a hot topic and refuses to wake from its anesthetic slumber, and pressure indicates that my catheter is not draining properly. My pleas to allow me to try to urinate naturally are accommodated with its removal. Bladder ultrasounds are conducted before and after I am toileted. Miserably uncomfortable, I desperately try and fail to channel a relaxing connection to the pelvic floor I was unaware of having. I also have performance anxiety. Humiliated, I beg the aides for privacy.

During a pleasant enough hall stroll with my mother, a urologist that I have never met and will never see again interrupts us to tell me that my trial is over. Common following surgery, my bladder requires rest and faces the risk of permanent damage without prompt catheterization. Scared straight and dejected, I ride another devastating wave and can barely muster the strength to walk the few steps back to my cell.

*   *   *

With my family evicted from my room, bright examination lighting illuminates me in my already ruinous state, now further splayed open, on my back with my legs bent and knees spread. I am alone with an experienced nurse who, try as she may, is unable to insert the catheter. I lose count, hope, and my mind.

A urologic oncology physician assistant is called in, assuring me that she has successfully performed thousands of like procedures, yet she continues to fail after multiple attempts as well. Poked and prodded to destruction with painful serial violations, my muscles are tense, vaginal tissues swelled, raw and angry, torn apart and ripped to shreds.

The last and best resort is the urologic oncologist on call. She arrives with skill and empathy, promising me that she will insert the catheter on the first try and she does. Having hurt me only to help me, the three women surround my raised bed and look down on my ravaged body. In the aftermath of a sympathetic clinical gang rape, I am in sheer agony.

In a final heinous act of care, I will be sodomized when my nurse returns to administer an enema. I beg her not to, cry, tell her I need to go to the bathroom (my rumbling digestive system arising in the nick of time). I am nauseous and on the verge of vomiting. Nonetheless, firm and determined in her professional ministries, she delivers a final violating treatment out of necessity. Utterly shattered, I cannot recover from the annihilation.

*   *   *

Kindly, my nurse brings me an aromatherapy treatment in the form of a small plastic pill cup with a lavender oil saturated cotton swab. Though it hardly proves amply soothing under the circumstances, I appreciate the thoughtful gesture, and the scent eases my derangement.

This unforgettable incident will be one of the most damaging and haunting that I face. Where the fuck was the morphine?!

*   *   *

Always bustling in energetically at some ungodly early morning hour, my hematologist oncologist monitors my progress despite my negligible consciousness. Low iron levels indicate anemia and I can't unsee the enormous shot filled with thick black sludge that will course through my veins.

With encouragement, he briefly shares his own cancer history and that of his beloved wife, who also had ovarian cancer. Still smitten, he shows me a picture of her. She radiates joy, is blonde and younger. He adores her.

Perhaps I remind him of her, and he visits me first on his rounds because he is anxious to see me. Or, perhaps he wants to distance the painful memory I evoke from the rest of his day. He will later confirm what I had immediately intuited.

*   *   *

Mummified, my abdominal bandages are temporarily removed

and I am asked if I would like to look. Repulsed, I refuse and turn away. My husband and mother investigate. My deprived father, who in recent years began lamenting that I never had children, spares himself from a too harsh reality and will never set eyes on my scar. We share a wicked sense of humor and I contemplate having the vile tumor swaddled in a clean baby blanket and delivered to his empty arms, in place of the grandchild that he will never have.

*   *   *

Ever the gracious hostess, my accepting and pleasing nature knows no bounds. My empty womb was generous to the brink of death. Polite and welcoming, a perfect repository for this tumor, however beastly and insidious it may be, efficiently laying waste to my unsuspecting body.

Displaying the most cordial and arcane hospitality, I have accommodated without protest an organic love child attempting to consume me from the inside out. An abomination, repugnant in its entirety. Filled with revulsion, I am disturbed to my core.

*   *   *

Amid smoke and ashes, the first sign of life as we knew it is when I request that an askew lampshade in my room be adjusted. I ask my mother to bring me the heirloom birthday ring I have designed for my elder stepdaughter's upcoming birthday. Noting a detail not to my specifications, I dispatch her back to the jeweler for timely action. I can't stop making things beautiful, I will be the fool rearranging furniture and art work as flames lick at my hands and my house burns to the ground.

My boundaries are set in stone. I take only one call from family, to reassure my younger stepdaughter, to discourage her from visiting, to spare her seeing me so dilapidated. Protecting one of my loving oldest friends from what I know will unnerve her, I instruct my husband in how and when to disseminate information. The only person I have informed directly of my plight is my close friend, our connection is so profound and genuine that we communicate telepathically. During a brief call I tell her that I will be discharged with a walker to our artistically curated home. For the first time post-surgery, and at the risk of hemorrhaging, I laugh with her, pained and euphoric.

*   *   *

Anticipating my release, a specialized nurse arrives to remove the CVC from my jugular. Grotesquely associating a slit throat with a bloody death, I find it both disturbing and comforting to have this vessel used as a portal, with open house injections and extractions sparing me the additional angst of a needle's puncture. To reduce the critical risk of bleeding and air embolism during the procedure, the head of my bed has been lowered below my heart and I follow breathing instructions. We spend an intimate 5-10 minutes together post-removal, while she applies constant pressure to the site. The scars on my neck will be a lasting reminder, lest I forget.

*   *   *

One of my favorite recovery nurses, along with an assisting nurse, attempts to prepare me for straight catheterized home care. Well enough desensitized with opioids to tolerate the assault, my urethra has retreated to Never Never Land, and despite earnest efforts by the three of us to locate it, she shan't be found. The last try involves me suggesting I sit on my nurse's lap to enable her to instruct me from behind. Layers of morphine and other narcotics enable me to endure the unsuccessful attempts with bizarre good humor, and we giggle at our foils. I am re-catheterized and will be sent home with a fixed Foley catheter for one week to enable my bladder to recover from the trauma of surgery, without the benefit of intravenous drugs and comedy.

*   *   *

I never anxiously await my hospital discharge. Wounded as I am, I have no faculties to operate on my own anymore. Too ruined, wasted and weak to stand on my own or dress myself, I am dependent and require assistance for nearly everything.

On day eight, with little desire to escape my confinement, I am released. Driving home, my husband is as emotionally pained as I am physically. I brace myself in the passenger seat against the searing pain that every bump or jostle delivers. With a white-knuckled grip on the car's grab handle, I will learn to float and ingest pain as I am shuttled from appointment to appointment. With every action driven by an extensive medical team directing my next move, it will be months before I will get into a car to go anywhere else, months before I will feel up to driving again. My sole purpose in life has become survival.

*   *   *

Generally poised and confident, I return to the sanctity of our condominium with little autonomy, in a residentially toxic cesspool that is sure to have been the trigger if my onset was stress induced. Ashamed and decrepit, I am hunched over a walker and dread being seen by extended family, friends or exceptionally nice and inconceivably nasty neighbors. For the first time in my life, I am pitiful.

*   *   *

Having left everything perfectly decorated for Christmas, I come home to masses of flowers. Deeply touched by so many thoughtful and generous deliveries, I am thankful yet overwhelmed. One enormous funeral-esque arrangement in particular makes me wonder if I have died. I ask that the blood red and icy white stunner be redirected to a nearby nursing home, where it is sure to be appreciated and enjoyed.

*   *   *

Unable to bathe in the hospital, I am desperately looking forward to cleansing myself. I anxiously await the purifying and restorative powers of our bathroom, now equipped with an unsightly shower seat.

Undressed, I see myself for the first time. Frankenstein, a monster, abdominally gutted, stapled together and bandaged. A pubic mullet and the fucking Foley, trailing from what's left of my vagina and strapped to my right thigh–invasive, uncomfortable and repulsive.

Even with assistance, the four-inch shower curb is a challenge to navigate, but I insist. Physically pleasured for an instant, I close my eyes and weep with gratitude as I become reaccustomed to the luxury of water and soap running through my hair and down my body. When I open my eyes, I see all the destruction and weep in horror. Waves of sheer terror wash over me, and I nearly collapse exiting the shower.

Convinced that I have dislodged the catheter, I gingerly make my way to our bed. In the fetal position, I call the hospital's emergency line within hours of being discharged. Reassured that all is well enough, I am tranquilized returning to our marital bed, feeling my husband by my side.

*   *   *

In shock and denial, I am impossibly hospitable. The day after my release, we have company for the holidays. At my insistence, the show must go on!

With significant apprehension, my husband and mother are tasked with removing my jugular bandaging. I believe that he has grazed my neck with scissors in doing so and fall into another fit of nervous and happy hysteria. I am the only one laughing maniacally.

My mother helps me dress and when my elder stepdaughter and I greet and hug, she cries and apologizes for her emotional reaction. Touched by her sensitivity, I hold her and stroke her hair. I release her from our longstanding end-of-life pact. Later, in an act of compassion and solidarity, my younger stepdaughter will cut and donate her pure thick tresses, her only practical vanity. My stepson will demonstrate empathy in many unexpected acts, thoughtfully checking in and delivering a dream weaver from Alaska. They will join forces with considerate care packages and treats to celebrate milestones. For the first time, it is clear to me that our unidealized family has grown beyond tolerance and function. Finally settled, we have again become unsettled, though now I feel the genuine bonds of familial love.

We make a homemade pasta dinner with our soon-to-be son-in-law and will braise lamb for a holiday lunch with the children. Our older grandson sweetly reaches up to pat my belly with both hands. In a quick panic, his mother gently stops him, though I can bear the discomfort and relish his affectionate touch. Our younger grandson is still in his infancy, contained, happy and playful. The boys will remain innocent and oblivious throughout my downfall, my worries are wasted.

*   *   *

My husband puts me to bed. Like a baby, I cannot get in or out without him. The slightest movement is agonizing and I fear that our house guests will hear me whimpering during the night. Constantly paranoid about the catheter bag filling, I go to the bathroom multiple times with my husband's assistance. Debilitated and demeaned, I have been diminished to requiring my lover to detach, empty, clean and reattach the vessel that voids my bladder. I was once dignified and lady-like.

My most basic bodily functions are now rooted in dread and loathing. Managing my digestive system is excruciating. It has become, and will remain, nearly unbearable. With tear jerking struggles to purge my bowels, I use senna tea, drugs and warm compresses for relief. Unable to sit or stand without assistance, for months I will count on a towel bar, mobility device or strong arm to bear my full weight and weakness.

*   *   *

After a week's respite, on Christmas Eve, a much-anticipated day has arrived when I meet my urologic oncologist to remove my despised catheter. Wracked with performance anxiety, I want my husband and need my mother, who potty trained me at six months by tethering me to a toilet shortly after my birth. During the procedure, attentive to romancing the doctor, I self-consciously notice that I haven't shaved my legs since before my hospitalization. Reduced to my infancy goals, I am flooded with relief at being able to naturally relieve my bladder. Hallelujah and good fucking riddance to Foley and the horse he rode in on!

The doctor connects with me compassionately, telling me that she is my age. Given the gravity of my cancer diagnosis, she recommends that I obtain a second opinion.

That evening, we make a brief appearance at our family's annual Christmas gathering. In the garage on the way to the car, I nearly collapse in front of the children, flush with embarrassment. I refuse to enter my sister-in-law's home with a walker to face my extended family and rely on my husband for support.

*   *   *

My right knee continues to buckle, and in addition to frequently collapsing only to be jarringly caught, I fall. The first time is entering the kitchen pantry, and I laugh and call out to my husband, assuring him that I am okay. I fall again in the garage and again in the bedroom, hitting my head and dangerously close to the large plate glass window. My husband is concerned and dead serious while I laugh my way through each fall, though the last one is especially painful, and I suffer the consequences for days after.

With multiple post-surgery collapses and falls, I narrowly avoid catastrophe and gain much medical attention. I meet with a physical medicine and rehabilitation specialist who tests the response in my right leg to no avail. I have absolutely no reflex in my right knee with manual or electrical stimulation and feel nothing at all when he uses safety pins to test the surface of my leg. Many evaluations by an array of fascinated experts will eventually lead to the unfortunate diagnosis of a femoral nerve injury and months of intensive physical therapy (though I have avoided irreparable damage).

*   *   *

Asked during appointments if I feel safe at home, I reply that I do. I am only subject to harm in the medical facilities where I continue to suffer inhumane and brutal treatments.

In a seemingly endless process, forty-four staples are removed. To carry myself to a terminable end, I request progress reports during the pinching and pulling. My souvenir is a long and jagged scar, running from the base of my sternum all the way down to my pubic bone. I am a decimated wasteland, lying on the bed awaiting the further violation of a pelvic exam.

I experience visual disturbances and chronic migraines and am convinced that the cancer has metastasized to my brain. My oncologist quells my worries and assigns me her detailed treatment plan.

I have survived surgery only to be awarded a chemotherapy regimen. Of all the brutal acts that those drugs will take on my body, I am immediately inclined to preserve my threadbare vanity above all else. My first question is if I will lose my hair.

*   *   *

In *The Ultimate Guide to Ovarian Cancer*, Benedict B. Benigno, M.D. ponders the treatment being worse than the disease. "One looks forward to surgery as a singular process. The process of chemotherapy is repetitive and carries with it intimations of mortality. There ensues a rage, the darkest rage, lightened by nothing. No matter how large and loving the family, a feeling of isolation and dissociation pervades all aspects of her life. Loneliness and aloneness become part of the daily routine. Surgery and the administration of chemotherapy are far easier for me than an attempt to keep so fragile a patient from dissolving and simply giving up. It represents the supreme moment of vulnerability and raises loneliness to an unspeakable level. …the secret is to turn adversity into triumph."

Physically and emotionally devastated, without energy or stamina, I have no ability to do the job for my oncologist and fear that I will fail her.

*   *   *

Determined to regain confidence with a plan, I enter a chemotherapy education meeting flanked by my husband and parents. Considering the infusion schedule, it appears that we can successfully work around our upcoming trips to Malta in February and a Baltic Sea cruise in April.

Gifting me momentarily with a sense of control, after a long pause my oncology nurse gently expresses her concerns regarding my access to qualified care should I opt to travel during treatments. She questions what services I will find on a miniscule island in the middle of the Mediterranean Sea, if I develop a therapy induced neutropenic fever and require urgent specialized medical attention.

Our plans will be canceled, we have been grounded. Under grave threat, my role is that of compliant spectator. No longer in the driver's seat, I am a passenger in my own body and completely dependent on my practitioners, whose skills are my only hope for salvation. I had no idea that to secure a chance at survival, I would be forced to relinquish my aspirations, my life.

*   *   *

Accepting a barbaric and archaic treatment plan requires implicit trust and a blind eye. I brace myself for the assault of six treatments, every three weeks, horrified by the medically choreographed dance between destruction and sustainment. Chemotherapy will viciously attack everything in its path, without discrimination and with cumulative effects. Overextending my capacities and mustering the will to accept the abusive cycle once, I will face it again, again, again, again and again.

In *Memoir of a Debulked Woman: Enduring Ovarian Cancer,* Susan Gubar describes how "War, which can be defended on ethical grounds, resembles chemotherapy because both set out to wreak massive injury, even if collateral damage may inadvertently be inflicted. In the contest or battle between chemotherapy and cancer, in which there can only be one winner and one loser, the supporting army on the chemo side should be comprised of valiant volunteers dedicated to 'a good war,' for the foe takes as its goal nothing but extermination."

My aversion to toxic drug cocktails cannot be countered with faith in their success rates. My prognosis is poor and even "gold standard" treatments are resisted by my genre of cancer. My only guarantees are lethal metastases or side effects that are patently worse than those produced thus far by the disease.

*   *   *

We are advised of chemotherapy contamination and contagions, practices and protocols. I will be tainted, further isolated physically and emotionally, in shame and embarrassment. Disgraced, I wonder how I can possibly tolerate direct administration and ingestion, if my diluted emissions from any and all orifices are so toxic and to be avoided by others at all costs.

I'm offered a chemotherapy port and spared the gory details. No one mentions the incisions at the base of my neck and upper chest, the insertion of a port, the catheter being tunneled under my skin, over my collarbone and into my jugular vein, how it will terminate in my superior vena cava, just above my heart. We do not discuss the long, bevel tipped needle that will slide through my skin, just as easily as through the silicone septum of my implanted port's reservoir, drawing blood and delivering intravenous medications and contrast solutions. Never mind about the constant reminder, clearly demarked above my right breast, or the related risk. No, thank you.

Against recommendations, I decline the intrusion in favor of IV administration.

*   *   *

A product of my Italian heritage, where we even have a term dedicated to aesthetic impressions (*la bella figura*), I don't discount the value of appearances. Proud and vain, a significant portion of my sense of self is tied to my image. I, however, do not participate in the hypocrisy of the comically conceited, toting the value of beauty on the inside while immersed in an inauthentic, modified and manipulated culture of ridiculous self-display. Amid grotesque social media and sexist advertising campaign norms, my conceits lie solely in recovering my intrinsic sense of self.

Following my husband's brilliant and empowering suggestion, my hair is cut into a short shag on December 30th. My dear stylist liberates me to enter the new year feeling chic and encouraged, with many compliments and assumptions that I am wearing a wig. Possibly mad, I experience phantom hair pain.

*   *   *

While the male is nobly designed to perform at any advanced age, the female is engineered for penetration and procreation.

Indelibly changed, from a lush tropical forest to a barren desert, I have been made less functional. My feminine core has been reduced to a road to nowhere, a dead end.

Unaware of the ramifications of The Change, in the seconds it took to remove my ovaries, surgically induced menopause has plunged me instantaneously into the deep end of a hormonal transition that would naturally occur later in my life and span a period of seven to ten years. In addition to directing menstrual cycles and all things childbearing, estrogen and progesterone affect skin, bones, muscle mass, blood pressure, cholesterol, brain function, inflammatory response and emotional reactions.

The full brunt of menopause, amplified by the physical and emotional repercussions of my conditions and compounded by adjunct steroid treatments, will lead to extreme hormonal chaos with no window to abatement. Risks prohibit the use of hormone therapy, and I will tolerate the effects for years, with no remedy or end in sight.

WAGING WAR

January 2020

"There are some things you learn best in calm, and some in storm."

Willa Cather

I witness the permanent unravelling of my beautiful life. Unhinged in my own skin, I occupy the skeleton and soul of a stranger, anchored to a body I don't trust and a deranged mind. I am outraged by my body's betrayals and by the violent assaults to save me. In ruins, my foundation has been demolished and I will never stand on solid ground again. My sorrow is immense and devours me.

I weep, beg to go back in time. Immersed in comparative thinking, I anguish in the before and panic in the now. Devastated by what I have become and the path my life is taking, I am unable to accept reality.

Shocked to be facing an impossible task, I can't let go. I simply don't know how. Helplessly suffering, I am inconsolable and mired in what I have lost and how likely I am to lose absolutely everything. Broken, I have come entirely undone.

*   *   *

With a history of wellness, I have no threshold for what my body can handle, for what is survivable.

I transition from tall, slender and toned to emaciated and skeletal in no time. At my most decrepit, my 5' 8" frame has wasted away to 112 pounds. Nipples are the only thing left of my scant breasts and my severely atrophied muscles showcase every bone protruding from my lax skin. Literally starving, I will know ravenous hunger for the first time. Havoc has been wreaked, and I wonder how much I can sustain before I expire.

I can no longer comply with my mother's long-standing dictate to stand up straight! My insides scream in protest when I extend or stretch my core from its wounded and protective shell. When I have been at rest and move, I feel constriction in my abdomen, the pulling and tearing of tissues that knit themselves back together being torn apart again. Abdominally disorganized, I know nothing of what has been taken away, what I am left with and where my remaining organs have settled.

*   *   *

Vulnerable to my own thoughts, panic rises in the still and I am rarely left alone. No longer a controlling administrator, confidently undoing, correcting, revising or walking away at will, my competence has been crippled. Unaccustomed to wallowing in misery, I am dejected and bewildered, flailing frantically for a lifeline to pull myself up, though I am impotent.

My husband is my most intimate companion, always grounded and certain. He will never falter, never leave my side, never shy away from physical or emotional challenges. My mother is a giver and provides comfort and compassion, she is always of service. I cry out for her when weeping uncontrollably in blind despair. Not understanding my primal need, my husband tries to console me himself and in doing so withholds my only cure. Facing death, I have been reduced to an infantile desire for the woman who birthed and nurtured me, her healing hands being the sole balm to sooth me.

*   *   *

Motivational passages promise that I can trust that as fast and far as my fear can travel, my courage will outrun it. I strain to hold the door to my past open, as if my old life is there waiting for me, yet I must muscle my way forward. Set down my grief for the life I intended to have but won't, focus my mind on the life I hope to have, commit to the present. Envision a tether of light pulling me towards a point in the distance, widening the bridge between my demons and me.

I am to consider all that I've outlived, my durability, adaptability and resilience. I am to walk, not crawl, towards my new life, my next life. I must imagine what might await me on the other side of this dark forest, the sun shining in a clearing.

*   *   *

I attempt to resume control with a calendar, noting and color coding my treatments. Ticking off the days, I will chart life on the inside and parole.

Not knowing what to expect and anticipating being bedridden (which I never am) I established standards for myself that I will proudly maintain with ease. My self-disciplines include:
- Prioritize wellness and invest in self-care without guilt.
- Brush/floss regularly.
- Keep your nails painted.
- Wear earrings and dress well.
- Be productive every day, no matter what.
- Never lose sight of your blessings, be gracious and grateful.
- Maintain your sense of humor.
- Be honest with yourself and others, ask for and accept help.
- Keep up with communications and focus on others.
- Practice mindfulness, stay rooted in the now.

*   *   *

Our community's wellness center is a supportive facility, dedicated to programs and services designed to strengthen, empower, educate and provide hope to patients with cancer and their families. Over the course of my treatments, I will offset difficult activities with those that are soothing and restorative.

One of my first acts is both awful and encouraging. My parents accompany my husband and me to a sad and comical wig fitting before I start losing my hair.

My lovely mother, from whom I inherited my style and vanity, will later accompany me to a Beautiful You presentation, where I am one of many inspiring and pathetic participants in varying stages of decay. She scolds me when I whisper to her that instead of taking notes, I am contemplating stabbing myself in the jugular with the pen that has been provided. I follow her directive to behave and volunteer to model for the make-up demonstration. A swag bag includes a gorgeous "Just Kissed" pink lip stain!

Indulging in a facial, I am driven to distraction by the technician's oversized latex gloves and wonder if she is protecting me or herself.

My mother and I attend a relaxation and meditation class substituted by an enthusiastic yoga instructor. From the ground, my tiny bird-like mama assists me as I attempt to crawl into positions and finally right myself. We seek a bright core of light that we never find and giggle. In this safe and nurturing space, I am reminded that I can still feel happy.

I prepare a therapeutic hot bath and adjust a collection of brass candlesticks. Immersed in the cocoon of warm water, I retreat to the womb, go back, start over. Deeply relaxed, I am jolted at the thought of my submerged incision and realize that I am likely breaking a rule, which I am.

*   *   *

My husband adds to his nursing duties, carefully following extensive pre- and post-infusion instructions to the letter. No longer dependent on my immune system, I have been prearmed with four vaccinations, delivered in pairs to both of my arms during a single session.

*   *   *

Entering my first infusion with fear of the known and unknown, I realize that my saviors are especially lethal when approaching me in specialized hazmat garb as a team, with secondary practitioners in tow to verify all drug administration details.

As meticulously as they dispatch the treatments, my body promptly protests round one. My liver values are out of range and will recover just in time for round two.

*   *   *

Bound and determined, I meticulously manage every infinitesimal opportunity to restore a life outside and inside my confines, to deliver and return a sense of civility to our compromised lives.

Actively seeking comfort, I will eventually establish a Chemotherapy Eve routine. On the evenings prior to my infusions, I undress and nestle into a soft robe. In-home massage therapy precedes a food truck's roasted chicken and slaw, enjoyed curled on the sofa in our den with a mindless TV show.

During each infusion, my husband and I are satiated in each other's company and my parents make a cheerful visit, as do a sympathetic nutritionist and social worker from the wellness center.

Impressing my team with my exemplary diet and resources, I strive to be a model patient, aiming for an A plus in a circle. Friendly as they are, kindness never concedes to medical care, and my requests to consume raw oysters, smoked salmon, sushi and blue cheese are always denied. Alcohol is strictly prohibited, though I have lost interest anyway. I will eventually succeed in negotiating a thimbleful of wine when I have a taste for it,

50

restoring cultural norms to our dinners.

I cling to the rare occasions when I am presented with a choice, requesting the ongoing care of my immediately favorite infusion nurse. With my second treatment onward, I opt for a convenient on-body injector of bone marrow stimulant to save us a return trip to the cancer center. The device is startling when it activates, and I assure our kindly neighbors that I am not a suicide bomber when the ticking starts during one of our visits.

*   *   *

My femoral nerve injury proves to be one of my most challenging deficiencies, requiring extensive specialists, evaluations and treatments.

Further evidencing my decline, my handicaps are made public. I will be fitted with a knee brace and begrudgingly graduate from a walker to a cane. Thoughtlessly bounding up and down stairs in my gazelle-like past, I am now reduced to elevators and an interminable process. For months, I will work towards taking stairs like a toddler learning to walk. With trepidation, I grip the rail with both hands and ascend or descend every tread with multiple tentative steps. My progress will be measured in the monumental accomplishments of using one hand on the rail instead of two and later taking steps one at a time.

*   *   *

On meeting my masterful physical therapist for the first time, post-surgery and pre-chemotherapy, I emulate a horse beyond repair and suggest that she take me out back and shoot me. She elects to not shirk her responsibilities, and we quickly develop a special relationship. Deeply connected, she will easily laugh with me during dozens of sessions. I set aside my despair, frustration and disgust with my limitations and enjoy our joyous release! She is invaluable, providing guidance, encouragement and healing in every visit.

Equally trained, gifted and dedicated, this incredible woman nurtures me back to wellness under the direst circumstances. Concerned and determined, she is intuitively sensitive to my needs and abilities. She handles me with careful consideration, knowing when I can tolerate weight-bearing activities in common areas and when, too weak from the repercussions of chemotherapy, I will need to be treated on the table in her private room with a closed door and dimmed lights.

The strength in her limbs and muscles make up for the weakness in mine, as she works with me to maintain the neurological connection that could be permanently lost in the year it will take my nerve to repair itself. With my husband's dedicated ancillary physical and emotional support, I will follow her extensive rehabilitation regimen, multiple times daily, over the course of many months. I give myself over to her with implicit trust, follow her recommendations and push myself to achieve goals. Under her care, my body works to heal itself.

*   *   *

With encouragement from my urologic and gynecologic oncologists and pressure from my parents, I seek an expert second opinion from the lauded department chair of a renowned university hospital, a scientist and physician highly specialized and respected in the field of ovarian cancer. Protected from survival statistics, I naively anticipate the meeting with confidence, seeking assurance. I dress for the occasion, wearing my mother's silk scarf with jewel toned peacocks. My husband, parents and I trek into the bedlam of a big city, through a seemingly antiquated facility, hordes of people and brusque staff, in a setting lacking all the luxuries I have come to expect.

We fill a small room, and in a tight corner I perch on the edge of a bed awaiting his visit. My entourage leaves standing room only. During the few minutes he spends in the room, towering over all of us, he summarizes my surgery and diagnosis. He notes spleen and femoral nerve complications, concurs with the recommended adjunct treatment plan and advises that relevant clinical trials are not available at this time.

Commensurate with general literature, he advises that stage IIIB ovarian clear cell carcinoma is a lethal disease, and that few patients can be cured. Following surgery and treatment, 1/3 of patients will have a response to chemotherapy with a longer survival period, 1/3 will have a response with a more rapid recurrence, and 1/3 may have limited response requiring additional therapy. Swiftly delivering the grim statistics that I had been spared, we have been schooled by the professor.

I don't recall him laying a hand on me, though he casts my future without hesitation. He advises that there is little I can do to affect my outcome. His report will state that he is unfortunately unable to provide me with the positive reassurance I am looking for, that there are few modifiable life/environmental factors that will improve my outcome, that we will see how I respond to adjuvant chemotherapy. From a safe distance, he looks down into my despairing eyes and says "We all have a destiny." With his fateful promise, my flame of hope has been expertly extinguished. Poof, gone, just like that.

*   *   *

Before we depart, my mother and I stop in the restroom and she hugs me, though my limbs are limp and we don't speak. Both petrified and numb, in my abandonment, I am unable to consider the effect this has on her or anyone else.

Unanchored yet again, I gaze out the car window seeing nothing, knowing that my life has passed me by. I am mute and there are no countering reassurances from my family. Not a single word is uttered by any of us during the long drive home. Every minute of deafening silence confirms to me that we have all heard him, his judgment has been delivered and received.

*   *   *

I later stare at his official report and see that no one has taken the time to fill in the personal details that I had provided on the extensive forms required prior to our meeting. Twenty-nine times, the words "not on file" take the place of answers that define me as an individual. He knows me only by name, date of birth and condition. I am nothing more than a high complexity patient.

The time we spent together is grossly overstated, though he has made the effort to diagnose me with significant anxiety. He recommends drug-based treatment, though I will not succumb to a dulled or deadened emotional existence, nor take advice from someone who has no idea who I am or what I need. He possesses such great knowledge of my flesh and so little knowledge of my spirit.

Traumatized and terrified, in mere weeks, my entire world has unraveled at break neck speed. Enduring unimaginable assaults, I have been split from stem to stern, physically and emotionally gutted and crippled with a nerve injury. I face the ravages of six poisonous chemotherapy cycles. And now, the likelihood that even if I muster the physical and emotional courage to survive all that, the cancer may only be held at bay before it consumes me, though I am just as likely to succumb to it without further ado. More probable than not, a recurrence nearly guarantees that I will die in short or slightly extended order. Even in a better-case scenario, we can only hope for a durable/longer remission. Anxiety is defined as anticipating adversity or misfortune which has yet to happen, yet am I not already living in a state of adversity and misfortune, without the additional burden of his prophecy?

Recognizing and respecting the professor's professional competence and responsibilities, I can't negate the value of his opinion because it doesn't suit me, nor do I begrudge him for plainly speaking the truth. However, under the circumstances, I also necessitate the gift of compassion. Perhaps extending an olive branch of humanity would be against his Hippocratic Oath, perhaps it was just a bad day, perhaps he didn't recognize my frailty. Though he hasn't hurt me, he has unknowingly done me great harm.

*   *   *

Raw and defenseless, I rue the recommendation and the cataclysmic meeting that has left me in a monstrous and intolerable state of chaos. I will be haunted infinitely by our short time together, reliving his dismal view and lack of confidence, seeing my future through his eyes. Were he a gambling man, there is no doubt in my mind that he would be all in, favoring his vocational calling for a win.

Impressively accomplished in research and scientific treatments, the patient care at this well-respected facility is not a good fit for me and I will never visit it again. Further injured by testing other waters, I return home to the warm embrace of my own clinicians and facilities.

*   *   *

In the midst of a lightning strike, a random act of terror, I seek clarity and peace, though there is no sign of it on my horizon. Desperate to remedy my ignorance with understanding and fear with certainty, I will continue to question nearly every medical professional that I encounter, pleading for my life. A root cause analysis and clear plan of action with defined and believable results would suffice. Blinded by the dark, I pursue light in promises that cannot exist.

I want what can never be offered, keep pressing for the

impossible and even go it alone. I obsess over factors and figures, identify what does and doesn't relate to me, ponder cause and effect, magical thinking, luck and karma. I look for meaning in the rubble that surrounds me and the comfort that reasons provide, finding nothing but ruin.

*   *   *

Jealousy is not in my nature, though I sin with stage envy. Greedy for a better prognosis and relieved that it's not worse, I covet stage I, II and IIIA, anything lower than IIIB. Anything curable, treatable without surgery, chemotherapy and permanent physical and emotional scarring. Anything free of the crippling promise of recurrence. Anything less deadly.

I've been told by a friend with dyscalculia that my odds don't sound bad, but statistics are heavily weighted against me and twisted, perverse, torturous thoughts come to me naturally. My bloodthirsty hunter's sights have been set and I am engulfed in terror as cancer plays Russian roulette with me. More than every other chamber of a pistol has been loaded with its bullets. Every single day, I wake to feel the cold steel pressed to my temple, and brace myself in breathless dread as the trigger is pulled.

When I challenge my oncologist with the professor's prediction, she hopes that I will perform much better than expected, given my personal factors and more limited disease compared to other patients in the cited statistics. Beleaguered by my incessant begging, she generously offers 50/50 survival odds. She reminds me that my risk of recurrence diminishes with time and that my chance of surviving a recurrence increases with time. Nonetheless, over a five-year period, while 70% of us will be dead and gone, nothing is guaranteed. I could be the 1% with the worst possible outcome or the 1% that outlives everyone else. She reminds me that ultimately, it does not matter what the statistics say. Odds are numbers, not sentences or promises.

Humbly, she does not hesitate to liken patient outcomes to independent means and measures. She recommends that I focus on my own journey, give this fight my best shot and accept whatever I can't change despite best effort. This will be the only way to find peace with a cancer diagnosis and the uncertainty it brings.

I am guided away from looking at fog banks and assuming the worst and encouraged to plan and invest in my immediate and short-term future, but I fear that I have already dodged my allotment of bullets. I am howling at the moon and lacking in lives left.

*   *   *

From the comforts of an executive chair, I pride myself on my skills dealing with difficult situations and crises. With limited skin in the game, I am well accustomed to leading with success, yet the fierce independence and drive that have served me so well personally and professionally have now become my downfalls. I am unable to relinquish control without duress, and relying on aids that don't work leads to continual frustration. In my greatest need, the abilities and resolve that I once trusted are rendered not only useless but detrimental to my healing. Incapable and ill-equipped, my tools are all wrong for this job.

Unable to administrate to life with cancer, I vacillate between manic highs and hopeless lows. In my grief, denial is dangerous, bargaining is a fruitless act, and acceptance is an unachievable goal. I despise my insecurities, weakness, and inability to conquer challenges with finesse and competence. I have no idea how to hang on and let go at the same time.

Reestablishing and maintaining my mental wellness is of critical importance, and I lack the ability to do so. Begrudging and skeptical, I humble myself by asking for help, not realizing that the emotional toll that cancer takes will require as much care as the disease itself, lest my body survive without my mind intact. Only later will I understand that internalizing my feelings without specialized resources to help me navigate through them would be akin to managing the disease without an oncologist.

*   *   *

In need of another specialist, my husband and I enter the office of a counselor at the wellness center who will change the course of our lives. Well prepared, I have devised a status management system, including check marks and highlights to map my progress. Tracking every grievance, I chart my maladies (woes) and identify my physical ailments and remedies. My emotional complaints are far more complicated to address and resolve (rather, to suppress and control).

All business and on a mission, within minutes of meeting her, I promptly deliver my notorious List of Woes. Haughty, I challenge her to fix me, to repair and restore the new me to the old me, to prove her resourceful value.

List of Woes

Disfigured

Damaged

Ruined

Broken

Suffering

Falling Apart

Anguish

Panic

Despair

Fear

Lack of Control

Hopeless

Loss

Insecurity
Devastation
Weakness
Pain
Helpless
Terror
Defeat
Death

*　　　　　*　　　　　*

My counselor takes me a step back, from the symptoms into the how and why. When my voice breaks, I immediately declare myself emotionally unstable and ask that she fix that too.

She asks the impossible of me—to live with cancer. The devastating truth is that my life before is irretrievable. Recovery is impossible and my new reality is the only path forward. Astounded and further sickened, I find her dictate unimaginable. I have no intention of accepting the unacceptable, of sharing my life's reins with a disease and my caregivers.

To add insult to injury, I am reduced from devising strategic global business plans to penning Dear Diary entries as if I am sixteen years old. Her assignments are not without merit, the journaling activities that I initially resist will become my bible.

*　　　　　*　　　　　*

The signs were all there in the before. Apocalyptic forewarnings during our last trip to Italy included an evacuation and diversion due to the discovery and defusing of a WWII bomb, the death of a barn swallow (one of my favorite birds) and an avalanche.

Intuitively gifted in the art of fatalistic thinking, numerous premonitions and verities secure my pending passing, including:
- My zodiac sign is Cancer.
- My hedonistic acts promise paradoxical consequences.

- I have long anticipated dying young.
- I recently purchased a sweater depicting a crab.
- My journal was a gift from someone who died of cancer, at the hospital where I was treated.

My counselor humors me, until she abates my fictitious convictions with cold hard facts and reminds me that intuition is only valid if I can do something productive with it. When I veer off track with intuitive magical thinking, citing *The Beautiful and the Damned* and *As I Lay Dying* on our bookshelf as a promise of what's to come, she releases her lasso to reel me in and guides me back into my lane.

*   *   *

In *Unimaginable, What We Imagine and What We Can't*, Graham Ward references Joseph Conrad's *Heart of Darkness*. Living in the midst of the incomprehensible and detestable, there are growing regrets, a longing to escape, powerless disgust, surrender and hate. "The nameless and invisible is more terrifying than any face given to evil. In trauma we are attracted to the very terror we're denying. Friction-free utopias flourish alongside apocalyptic fantasies… Both are imagined states governed by death." It's our imagination that wants soothing.

My counselor will present me with an interesting dilemma. I am asked to imagine meeting her on the street in the before, as innocent strangers. She can tell me what I will soon face, if I want to know. I immediately do, because I would do things differently, catch it earlier, stop it, save myself! She interrupts my path to redemption when she tells me that in this scenario, I can do none of that because I cannot control the outcome. Everything that has happened will still happen. The only difference is that I will live with knowing what's to come, impotent to change it. I ponder that damning weight for only an instant. Engaging and charming as she may be, I wouldn't stop

60

to chat. I wouldn't want to know.

*   *   *

An equally formidable force, my counselor will not hesitate to challenge me, to enlighten me, to spur my growth. She warns me against latching on to the unchangeable past or unknowable future, to evaluate how those thoughts serve me. She firmly directs me to reality, trains me to endure hardships and to navigate my course. To accept that people who care want an active role in my life, under any and all circumstances. She is even able to guide me into tolerance territory, and I am by nature exceptionally intolerant.

Immensely grateful, I feel my lost identity being found and saved. My counselor will be the most instrumental person aiding navigation in this discomfiting new world, she is our captain. With or without direct contact, I will internalize her views and lines of questioning. She will forever be my voice of reason, guiding me through life as it is.

WOE IS ME

February 2020

"He who fears he shall suffer, already suffers what he fears."
Michel de Montaigne

Malta dates back to the dawn of civilization. Marking the islands' golden Neolithic period, remains ironically include mysterious temples dedicated to the goddess of fertility. My family will not spend this month exploring those grounds, we will instead mourn our losses.

Living breath by breath, I discount conversations regarding future trips, as if I will recover and we will go back to the life I have been forced to abandon. Our world as we knew it has come to an end. I have little faith, and I worry about what the future holds. All I see is black.

Perpetually stunned and in shock, my mind is incapable of processing my reality and I drift away. Playing possum, I sit staring. Gone baby gone, disassociated from my body, mind and life. My husband asks where I go, calls me to come back to him. I am not me, I am nothing. I feel nothing, I have nothing to bring back home. I am lost, irrevocable, I have flown the coop.

*   *   *

As I begin to lose my hair, I gain Lady Macbeth like madness. During the light of day, I am determined to hold out for as long as I can. For the sake of my appearance, I will tolerate the period of loss as long as there are no publicly visible signs of shedding or thinning. In the shadow of evening, in panicked frenzies, I stand at the bathroom sink pulling my hair out. In a fury, I lose more of my mind with every strand. My husband tries desperately to pull me away from the mirror, threatens to shroud them all, but I cannot abandon facing the horror. Obsessive, I fight back when he attempts to redirect me. Maniacal, I cannot stop and come further unhinged, hair by hair, in sheer hysteria at the mass exodus.

Succumbing to the poisons of chemotherapy, I am stripped of the last vestige of who I was. I am left with no barrier between the truth and me. There will be no escape.

*　　　　*　　　　*

Terrified, humiliated and eventually resigned, I wait two long weeks to bring the process to a close. Aggravated and not wanting an audience, I reject my mother's request to participate in my shearing. This is no celebratory occasion.

On Super Bowl Sunday, my dear stylist comes to our home to shave my head and to restore a portion of my lost sanity. We have a personal connection, and she is kind enough to gift me with an act that I am sure pains her. I sedate myself prior to her arrival, to spare her the additional duress of my unfiltered emotions. I sit on a stool in front of the bathroom mirror and watch her take clippers to my scalp. At the end of the process, we are relieved when we discover my well-shaped cranium, and I have been liberated!

Real or phantom, I experience physical discomfort from my hair loss. My head on the pillow is sensitive, needling and prickly. Many months later, I will have growing pains.

*　　　　*　　　　*

My pathetic act of empowerment robs me of my last shred of dignity. With my bald or covered head, I have lost all autonomy, and my disease and battle are on display.

I learn about cooling caps too late, though imagine that my future self would not opt to endure additional suffering at her own hands, for a temporary lifeline to ruinous vanity. She would instead empower herself, without hesitation. With a rigid backbone, she would face the godforsaken mirror and look herself unflinchingly in the eyes. With shears in her steady hand and a guttural "fuck you" to fear, she would take control.

*   *   *

Inauthentically costumed, I am an actor in a play and know myself even less on a false stage. I don a wig only on rare occasions, seeking comfort in the inconspicuous barrier it provides but finding it uncomfortable to wear and nerve wracking. Vividly imaginative, I anticipate a gust of wind alighting wigs, hats and scarves to the street as I stand on the sidewalk exposed, naked and mortified. I develop cat-like reflexes, quickly righting and cursing any displacement.

Showers continue to be volatile. I compensate the trauma of facing my ruined body with holistic acts and thrill in the most miniscule authorities. Spared the chore of shaving my legs, I remove my razor from the shower and a visual reminder with it. Unhindered from the tasks of washing, conditioning, drying and styling my hair, I spend time perched on a stool, ministering to my depleted skin and nails with organic lotions and potions.

My angelic massage therapist tells me quietly at the end of our next session how beautiful I am...still...on the outside.

*   *   *

Following recommendations, we enter genetic counseling and testing as a progressive family. Another Pandora's Box opens as I contemplate the risks I face of developing breast and colon cancer. Further dejected and convinced of positive results, I visualize an even more dismal future. On the off chance that I survive ovarian cancer, I ponder if I would rather know and be proactive or again discover another cancer crisis, too late.

I do not accept the genetic counselor's call when it comes because I am busy investing in my future. We are with our cherished jewelers designing heirloom earrings with my great-grandmother's gold chain. I choose to be present, recognizing the rare times that I can elect to decline intrusions. When I return the call, late that Friday afternoon in the nick of time, the counselor's somber tone of voice is promising. In a memorable lesson in my poor intuitive skills, I learn that I am free of all genetic mutations and am positively elated with relief. I soar, though quickly sink. Without reason, I have nothing to grasp onto in this random abyss.

*   *   *

Perhaps imaginative, faithless individuals suffer more acutely at the hands of destiny. Our artistic passions make us more prone to an active imagination, leading us to amplify and extend our suffering by visualizing all the mechanics behind, in and ahead of it in gross detail. Affective forecasting invites us to play psychic, predicting future perceptions and feelings. We spend more time anticipating than engaging in events, and given that the threat of hurt and actual hurt are experienced the same way, we are distressed at rest, when nothing is actually happening.

Pema Chodron shares an inspiring perspective about a young warrior at battle with fear in *When Things Fall Apart*. On opposing sides, the warrior and fear exchange dialogue regarding how their battle may be lost or won. Fear wins by completely unnerving its opponent, to the point where it drives action. The warrior may listen, respect and even be convinced by fear, but wins by rejecting its direction.

If we don't explore the recesses of every fear-based thought that arises, and embark on the chain reaction that follows, if we don't train in withstanding that disconcerting energy without getting snared in by the drama, then we will always be afraid. Living with uncertainty and giving up hope that insecurity and pain can be exterminated will make way for the courage required to not panic in the midst of chaos, to relax in the groundlessness of a situation. Fear is simply a component of our imagination, and we fuel its power or defeat.

*   *   *

Hell bent to hold on, I arrange my husband's annual birthday adventure at a nearby country inn. Miserable with digestive issues, I put on a brave face, fearing this will be our last trip. Determined, I push through the winter snow and ice with my cane as we slowly stroll along the farm road. My husband builds a fire in our cabin, and I am captivated by the flames. Physically comforted by tea, my attention shifts to our compromised future, and I am awash in devastation. Pathetic, broken down and ugly, I loathe myself in the mirror but pull through with costume and makeup design. I rally for an intimate dinner in the property's historic general store. Leaning over the candlelit table into our conversation, I become positively hysterical imagining how flammable my wig is and the havoc that would ensue if it caught fire! Our laughter is exhilarating, releasing a rare surge of healing positive endorphins.

A Sunday snow storm blankets our long drive home, and I am plagued by searing abdominal pain. Convinced that my remaining organs are in the process of prolapsing through my severed abdominal muscles, an emergency call with my oncologist that evening is reassuring. I am only experiencing piercing post-operative muscle spasms.

*   *   *

Embarking on infusion three of six, I track a halfway milestone marker and visualize an end in sight. At the cancer center, I assess members of my tribe…wonder what my compatriots are in for and size them up. I presume that if they feel well enough, they do the same. If so, my age and older husband must make for good fodder. I discount this as human nature, though maybe we're just invading each other's privacy without malicious intent.

We are imprisoned, inmates in this sect, enslaved to the same club and cult. On the street, we recognize one another easily enough, sensitive to the signs. Scars, dressings and appendages take the place of prison grade tattoos. The nearly ignorable impression on the upper right chest wall of a port and demarcations that those in the know see. The shell-shocked aura of the wounded and defiant.

*   *   *

Victims connect in companionship and compassion, uniquely able to relate. Cancer survivors tend to unite, in support and awe of one another's courage and resolve. Mitigating my own anguish, it deeply pains me to witness theirs. I have moments of debilitating empathy, then sink into pits of self-despair, anchoring myself to the suffering and outcome of others, terrified that their current or recurrent story will be mine.

Conversely, I callously assess how many badges they have earned, internally discounting many well-wishing "me too" promises. Other conditions are either much better or much worse, though I imagine them linking me to failure either way. I track my age, prior health, lifestyle, diagnosis and treatments. Every detail puts things on par to enable me to validate or invalidate claims that I will be fine, or that someone knows what I am going through, or how I feel. Someone else surviving has little to do with whether I will, until I consider statistics or choose to form a magical link. Unable to control my emotional response, I coldly disassociate, trying to survive.

I'm not like them. I don't belong in this setting, I never will.

SICK AND TIRED

March 2020

"Be aware of the temporary nature of pain. The things that wound us don't last forever unless we are determined to lengthen their echo. If we do not wallow in pain, and instead limit ourselves to experiencing it, the pain will gradually fade, and we will be left with a learning experience."

The Book of Ichigo Ichie

Despondent and isolated, I am wrecked from the inside out. In acts of physical and emotional intimacy I am dull and mildly disengaged. I am numb and hurt, devastated and detached, violated and tender. I am hollow, empty, spent.

Utterly sick of myself, I detest my failures, my incompetence. I face moments of helpless rage, especially at nightfall, when I prepare for bed and see in the mirror who I have become. Three months of twice daily heparin injections have distressingly led to extensive bruising, contusions and cystic nodules in the meager tissue behind my sharply boned hips. We celebrate my transition to a blessedly oral anticoagulant treatment and my husband's freedom from his heinous ministries.

Along with a now irrelevant cowlick, I have inherited my mother's and grandmother's situational insomnia. My sleep is disrupted, and my life is a nightmare with no waking reprieve. There is no hiding from this merciless illness and little hope that I will succeed in securing my future. I want to abandon myself but cannot escape.

*   *   *

Unaware of the temporary nature of physical and emotional pain,

I work desperately to regain my sanity, to resolve my despair. Perpetually nervous, worried and stressed, I play games with language, try to brainwash myself, look for the magic and silver linings I don't believe in and abhor.

Sympathy
Interest
Charity
Kindness
&
Treats
Inspiration
Riches
Encouragement
Demonstration

Still madder than hell, I furiously seek positive offsets to my misery.

Food
Education
Dedication

Understanding
Prayer

*   *   *

Despite our authoritative planning, saving and investing, we have failed to guarantee our physical security. Known and well-defined threats now root reasonable action in accepting that there are no guarantees in life under any circumstances. Focusing on what is real, I challenge myself to maintain short term focus and to celebrate small and all milestones. I coach myself to embrace the opportunity to be stronger and dig deeper, to be positive and live well.

My spirits rise when I find my footing and I feel revived. The same strength that has brought me to this moment is still inside me and will accompany me wherever I am led. With trepidation, I imagine that if anyone can survive, I can. With determination, I imagine that if anyone can survive, I WILL!

*   *   *

I am in hiding from the masses. Ruined, vulnerable and wanting to be remembered intact, I avoid exposure and curious onlookers. After a period of social abstinence, my first outings are fraught with tension. I dread surrendering my autonomy. People may know or not know, care or not care. People may ask, acknowledge or say nothing at all. The impact of any of these scenarios is more inconsequential to me than the limitations I have imposed on myself. For insecurities that hold no real threat, I rob myself and my family of small acts of normalcy. The only way to empower myself is to take action or to choose not to take action, consciously.

In a bold act, I dare to arrange a lunch outing with my husband and parents. While apprehensive and nervous, I push myself to brave action and wear a colorful hat. (Earth angels gift their handiwork to cancer and wellness centers. When I am too shy to pull from the basket, my mother is my partner in crime, retrieving my favorites.) As we exit the restaurant, I receive a compliment from a hip chef who enjoys knitting! He unknowingly energizes me with courage.

*   *   *

Noting another flaw in my brutalized body, the veins in my forearms are visibly tracking from my wrists to my elbows, and I ponder the dangers of blood poisoning. After sleeping on it, I spend the first Sunday of the month communicating with my oncology nurse and visiting urgent care and the hospital.

The urgent care staff is out of their element and my parents join us at the ED, where we experience our first memorably intimate introduction to COVID. The masked staff indicate that this far away virus is actively invading our safe place, though we are still oblivious to the deadly pandemic that is well poised to rage globally at the expense of many millions of lives. Aware of the mortal risk posed by the virus and my severely compromised immune system, they recommend that I wear a mask.

Perplexed emergency practitioners coordinate with my oncology team. They bustle about exploring, identifying and developing a treatment plan. In protest to the barrage of IV chemotherapy, my veins have thrown up a white flag in surrender. I am diagnosed with phlebitis and serpentine supravenous hyperpigmentation, and a heavy-duty round of antibiotics is added to my drug regimen. In the bizarre and rare, my body knows no bounds.

*   *   *

Headstrong in staying the course, I take the hard path and continue to destroy my vascular system in the process. When complimented on how well I am looking, with immediate shame and regret, I perversely display my arms to my outer circle, pointing out heroin addict tracks on my right forearm and the pattern on my left forearm that looks distinctly like a rabbit.

*   *   *

My fourth infusion is hateful and exhausting, though my vascular system holds out, just barely. My oncology nurse, whose conservative care I trust and whose tender approach I appreciate, steps in to save me from myself. With only two treatments left, I must choose an alternate administration method to spare my veins from additional and permanent damage.

Profoundly disappointed in my most recent setback, I still cannot bear to have a chest port. The thought of another invasive attack and unnatural attachment, visibly embedded under the surface of my skin, is intolerable. I opt for the perhaps worse alternative of a peripherally inserted central catheter (PICC), with the same end result.

Anesthetized, I undergo a procedure to have a thin flexible tube inserted into the vein in my upper right arm and threaded into my superior vena cava. I am spared needles but uncomfortable and hugely agitated. Repulsed at my appendage, half in me and half out of me, it is physically distressing and rarely ignorable. With daily shower protection managed by my husband, weekly flushing and dressing managed by the cancer center, and removal extended from my last treatment to my first post-treatment CTs (anticipating disease and extended treatments), it is a constant reminder of my now tethered life. I step forward only to be pushed back, leashed to a disease, to drugs, to institutions, to clinicians, to everything I never had and never wanted.

*   *   *

I anguish in evidence of the new me, hideous and damaged beyond repair. Every shower is a drama and my husband continues to threaten to remove or cover mirrors, to tack me with horse blinders. I rebel in a fury, holding tight to my reflection and reality. It is impossible to look away.

Our counselor suggests taping messages of affirmation to the mirror and I laugh, as if I didn't have enough anxiety without the interior design disruption of tacky sticky notes and clutter. I will later relish tearing that bathroom apart and having it rebuilt. I will watch the destruction and take a crowbar and hammer to the tiles myself after our contractors leave for the day. Like me, the superficially sound surface when breached unearths structural issues invisible to the naked eye. To renovate, to correct, to rebuild, the base requires total destruction. All layers will be stripped away, ripped out and disposed of to clear the way for something sound. Our daily utilities will be served with function and form, perfectly conceptualized and executed. Now a place of horror, this room will eventually become a place of healing.

*   *   *

Madness, sheer apocalyptic madness… Historically, only one in three generations experience a global pandemic. The realities of COVID are now being laid bare. Battling my own deadly conditions with a compromised immune system, a fiendish virus threatens to destroy me, my familial and medical communities, and the world in its entirety. Our lives are spinning even more cataclysmically out of control, the weight is nearly unbearable.

Unforgettably, my oncologist leans in to look me intently in the eye when she tells me point blank that if I contract COVID with cancer, there is nothing she can do for me. She instills me with permanent defenses and I become fiercely protective of myself and others. I will carry her warning with me, always.

Never a germaphobe, I become hypersensitive to the spread of disease. I despair at the selfish actions of societies in crisis, at the gross ignorance and inconsideration of the homicidal individuals who transmit the virus without regard. We begin a nearly agoraphobic existence.

*   *   *

Alone and at risk, my carefully constructed support systems crumble, leaving me further deflated, stressed and threatened. Isolated, I will bear treatments and face ongoing medical interventions without familiarity, without distraction, without reassurance. Without the few comforts that I held dear.

I fear life and limb with a virus that we know little about. Answering screening questions adds to my distress, COVID symptoms mirror the effects of chemotherapy. With everyone under constant scrutiny and on edge, my restricted appointments are more clinical. I am robbed of giving and receiving physical affection, of smiles and telling facial expressions. The view to humanity has been obscured, we are at war with ourselves.

*   *   *

Awaiting my first treatment in the cancer center without my husband by my side, I watch an elderly man in a wheelchair cry, pained over the loss of his wife. I wonder if he is without family, what ill he is facing, who will comfort him and what his plight will be. I want to go to him, to hold his hand, to tell him how sorry I am, but I don't. I can't. In a setting with so many high-risk patients, stringent protocols prohibit our contact.

The muscles surrounding my throat throb, and I cry in solidarity with the widower across the room from me. Alone in that moment, we feel no love, no connectivity. My heart breaks into a million little pieces, piled up right next to his. We blow away.

I endure my solitary fifth infusion, treated to a room with a pond view.

*   *   *

My Lutheran paternal grandmother, who lived just shy of celebrating her 104th birthday, believed that there was nothing to fear in death. Fear lies in what may precede death. My Catholic maternal grandmother, who ironically lost her ironclad fortitude in her later years to a peaceful if demented mind, would chant *"fede, speranza, carità"* (faith, hope, charity), as well as *"il gatto sul tetto che scotta"* (cat on a hot tin roof). Her longstanding missives were *"Forza!"* (strength), *"Coraggio!"* (courage). In life and in memory, these admirable matriarchs have always been good guides.

*   *   *

My devout mother is not churchgoing, though prays inclusively and without prejudice daily. My wandering father founded his own unincorporated religious sect, Budu (marrying Buddhism and Hinduism, as he saw fit). Many years ago, he presented his own set of Thou Shall commandments one morning during a family breakfast in China. Though tragically lost, we hope to unearth his paper trail one day.

Both understanding and judgmental, my parents continue to circle back to my faithlessness and how I may garner peace of mind, though I will not be coerced or convinced.

Perhaps they seek comfort in my salvation, think that if I believe I can survive, I will. That I can omnipotently change the course of a disease that I never welcomed and can combat, but will never control. That without hope, I will secure my future, fall victim to the scourge that claims more lives than not. I can imagine them bemoaning my defeatist attitude if I don't make it, thinking that I sealed my own fate. That I chose to give up, to succumb, to fail, to die.

*   *   *

Respecting religion and the faithful, I do appreciate the bestowal of blessings and am never offended by beliefs that are different from mine. Comforted by all layers of protection, no well wish goes unnoticed or discounted. It all matters to me.

*   *   *

While I may be faithless in the biblical sense, I am as certain in my beliefs and convictions as the most religiously devout. I skirt the sin of idolatry by forcing and pretending no religious or faithful affinity. Despite my Catholic primary schooling, I call out to God only in ecstasy and agony.

As a liberal free thinker with conservative ideals, my constitution is generally based in optimistic realism. I find no solace in releasing my trials and tribulations to a greater being that I do not know and cannot imagine. There will be no divine intervention (unless I gratefully stand corrected). I seek serenity in a better believable point of view or outcome.

Though my creation and afterlife theories are strictly scientific, I do believe in miracles. My miracles swing wildly to both ends of the pendulum...

ENDLESS BATTLES

April 2020

"Only to the extent that we expose ourselves over and over to annihilation can that which is indestructible be found in us."

Pema Chodron

The timing is perfect. I will complete wrecking ball treatments in the spring, during a month of rebirth.

The chemical eradication, my only hope, will leave me alive for now but destroyed. I subsist with flu-like fatigue, watering eyes and a two-week twitch, a runny nose that causes me to sniff like a cocaine fiend, oral irritation and a metallic taste that I cannot displace. (A film will be painstakingly scraped from my teeth by a dental technician, when I am finally able to risk an outing for standard maintenance.) Toxicities escape darkly from the pores of my skin. Muscle and joint aches in my legs and feet, worsening neuropathy, and fingernail sensitivity all evidence my poisoning. Cell by cell, I am dying.

*   *   *

We have not set sail to explore the Viking's homelands, though COVID lessens my burden of having robbed my family of the life we intended to have. Our explorations will be close to home and we will spend an entire year noticing the miniscule seasonal changes that we would have missed. Having always thrived stone-cold sober on an average day, my husband and I relish the ties that bind us to the life we loved, still. Coffee in the parlor, being together at home, nice meals and reading are our sacred and unspoiled pleasures.

While hibernating contentedly within my inner circle, I am also emotional, frustrated and tense. In a single day, I start out strong, productive, appreciative and high, only to shatter by evening and hit rock bottom.

∗   ∗   ∗

My treatment plans are familiar, though I cling to my favored nurses like an insecure child. For every cycle, I tolerate the before, during and aftermath, recuperating just in time to do it all again, though with fewer faculties due to each treatment's venomous and cumulative effects. I face my sixth and final infusion, battered for the last time and alone.

My conditions are both compounded by my femoral nerve injury and aided by my rigorous daily physical therapy regimens. I religiously follow recommended diet, exercise and activity directives. I gulp oceans of water to flush toxins from my system. I embrace little victories and celebrate my lashes living to die another day, though they finally give out too.

∗   ∗   ∗

Tornados by nature prefer the path of wide-open plains, where they can sweep through the land unhindered. My terrain is one of peaks and valleys. I skirt the eye of the storm, nearly destroyed. Bracing tempest after tempest, amid debris and devastation, my capacities to recover are limited and there are funnel clouds as far as the eye can see, threatening, brewing. A professional forecast predicts that they will touch down again, and in short order, with deadly force. I cannot escape the vortex.

∗   ∗   ∗

The relief of completing my last brutal chemotherapy cycle is promptly replaced by the terror of recurrence. Making the ultimate investments for a fleeting chance at survival, it's taken everything I didn't know I had to survive surgery, to survive chemotherapy, yet I have earned no respite. I must pull from spent physical and emotional resources to manage and survive the aftereffects and ongoing risk. With my graduation to surveillance mode, I bear the weight of the world.

While my fans cheer my accomplishments and milestone, I am broken down in every sense and fighting to muster the strength to continue what will be a lifelong effort to keep disease at bay. I may smile, raise my glass, and toast to please them, but I have not been liberated. I am hyperaware and on edge, waiting…

*   *   *

I ponder the details of recurrence and how and when it may kill me. In my mind, it is catastrophic. In my nurse's mind, things will never unfold as horrifically as they did before. Caught at onset and treatable, on again off again chronic disease promises to systemically gnaw away at me, closer to the bone every time.

We laugh when I ask if they will dispose of my body in the examination room's wall-mounted hazmat bin, though I'm serious and need to voice my deep, dark concerns. Many times, things are not quite as bad as I have imagined them to be and I am consoled, if only slightly.

*   *   *

It's impossible to cast my future. I can't frontload every scenario with an agenda and preparedness for eventual outcomes. There are millions of ifs and no plans of action can be made when we have yet to identify the exact problem. In a best-case scenario, I will remain disease free for the rest of my long life. Alternately, I will just up and die. Though, that might not be the worst-case scenario. An infinity of more realistic scenarios exists, and the ones I most fear are in those likely shades of gray.

In *The Perfectionist's Guide to Losing Control: A Path to Peace and Power*, Katherine Morgan Schafler explains how, with little control over the world around us, we placate fear with a false sense of security in guaranteed conclusions that we invent. "There are too many factors at play, factors you cannot possibly foresee, for you to ever be able to successfully manipulate every outcome in your favor. If you can't let go of your attachment to the outcome, you will spend your life trading one fear for the other. Fear-based lifestyles are a perpetual scramble, a dizzying loop, a ring of fire." If we shelve control, we can redirect our energy into facing our fears without intimidation. Simply put, control is the antithesis of power.

*   *   *

Needing company in chaos and gifted in the art of seduction, I frequently attempt to lure my resolute husband in. When I lay out an array of worst-case scenarios, he calmly and stoically redirects me to the moment and refuses to react to my hypothetical tragedies. Withholding validation heightens my hysteria, and I reach deeper into my bag of tricks. Stubborn, I keep at it while he remains equally firm in his resolve to deal only with what is. Clearly, he either a: doesn't grasp the magnitude of risk; b: doesn't care; c: cannot imagine the unimaginable; or d: all of the above.

While he refuses to succumb to my advances and join me in my torturous exercises, he does not hesitate to engage in optimistic assumptions. Much to my chagrin, he picks up where our lives left off and dreams up trips, seemingly oblivious that he will more likely than not be widowed by me.

I pity his naivety and contemplate laying out a handsome suit for him to wear to my funeral. A vintage astrological pocket square will appropriately complete his attire.

*   *   *

Historically a realist, I now crave time machines and symbolic promises. When I discover a vintage book titled *The Unicorn* by Anne Morrow Lindbergh, I read a poem that moves me to my core. "The Unicorn in Captivity" describes the captive mythological creature, winded and spent, collared and tied. He could shatter his prison wall, escape them all. He could prove his liberty, but does not choose, for he would lose. In contemplation stilled and acceptance filled, looking on, from wall and bars, to an infinity of sky and stars. Wild and tethered, the unicorn lives in captivity, yet free.

*   *   *

All is not in fact lost. Below the layers of damage, some vestiges of the character that I recognize survive, convictions intact. I'm not disposed towards bitterness, to clinging to life's wrongs for masochistic comfort. In sickness and even more so in health, I see women enveloped in resentment, giving off an aura tangible enough to be felt from a distance. That I will never do, I refuse. It has never been me, and it will never be me. I will find myself, albeit kicking and screaming, and pull myself up to stand tall above my grievances.

*   *   *

Called without cause, I face an enigmatic warlord. Cancer is not evil so much as it is entirely self-serving and vastly successful in its pursuits. While I offer it no warm embrace, fighting an unconquerable force is always futile, and hatred corrodes only the vessel in which it's contained. In a more realistic and positive bent, I will indeed fight, though not against cancer. I will fight for myself, by learning to live with it.

With a grounded sense of self and a whip in hand, I will be lorded over by nothing and by no one.

WHY NOT ME

May 2020

"Not everything that is faced can be changed. But nothing can be changed until it is faced."

James Baldwin

One dose away from total toxicity, my body has been abandoned in an utterly ruinous state. We shuttle to various appointments on a nearly daily basis, though my husband can only accompany me to the facility door and await my return. With visitor restrictions in place, I am further isolated, traumatized, terrified and alone.

*   *   *

Sunday, bloody Sunday… Extreme swelling in my left knee and ankle lead me to another holy day ED visit. The hospital is my church, the doctors there offer salvation from the ones who have had no choice but to subject me to their satanic interventions. An ultrasound relieves my nurse's suspicion of deep vein thrombosis, and I am diagnosed with lymphedema, another uncurable ailment that will require extensive treatments and lifelong management. One more blasted thing.

*   *   *

With no evidence of disease in my first post-treatment CTs, I am awarded a state of clinical remission and charged with both monitoring my body for signs of recurrence and living as though the cancer will never return.

Our first brush with liberty is inhibited by a raging pandemic. After six months dedicated primarily to my survival and care, I hoped to relieve my burdened family, to restore us, to make us whole again. Finally able to imagine living my legacy, we remain threatened and imprisoned.

I wonder how much time I have left, and if I will spend my stint prior to recurrence stagnant instead of making more memories. I wonder if we will have a future, another trip, another dinner party, another connection to life beyond our current constraints.

*   *   *

My hematologist oncologist marvels at my progress and releases me from PE treatment. Guilty of surviving, I ask about his wife. He lost the love of his life to the disease, as did my dentist. Two young women, married to doctors, wiped off the face of the earth. Wondering how he pushed through his pain, how he navigates his loss and loneliness, I am paralyzed by the lump in my throat and cannot speak. I will continue to find too many connections in our small community. The statistics will never make sense to me.

*   *   *

Two days later… Without a hand to hold, a nurse prepares me for my PICC line removal and scares the hell out of me by telling me to bear down. When I question her, she assures me that women can handle the procedure, it's the men that tend to balk and faint. Perhaps those women have borne children. Balking a bit though not fainting, I hold my breath to reduce the risk of air embolism and adverse events—ischemia and/or cardiac arrest.

*   *   *

Three days later… When instructed to change into a hospital gown for the removal of my IVC filter, I meekly ask permission to keep my knit hat on. Slightly sedated, I feel nothing but I know everything and tears stream down my face. The operating room nurse asks if I am okay, and I lie to reassure her. How can I possibly be okay?

*   *   *

In *Everything Happens for a Reason (and other lies I've loved)*, Kate Bowler writes "I had to face the fact that my life is built with paper walls, and so is everyone else's. It is a hard thought to accept that we are all a breath away from a problem that could destroy something irreplaceable or alter our lives completely. We know in life that there are befores and afters. I am asked all the time to say that I would never go back, or that I've gained so much perspective. And I tell them no, before was better."

Like Bowler, I will never giftwrap my cruel fate, it is no present. I have lost too much of myself and gained an education that only a masochist would welcome. No one sees the physical and emotional scars that I live with. Even under the best circumstances, I will never be quite right. The old me has been exterminated.

*   *   *

My crew is an exceptionally supportive lot and minister to me with loving and magnanimous consideration. They want me to be well. Some even declare emphatically that they know I will be okay, with the confidence I am unable to obtain from my skilled medical team. With admiration, I have been told that I was strong when I was weaker and more incapacitated than I have ever been, leaving me both insulted and encouraged. Their hearts are always in the right place and they are well-intentioned, but I'm a realist and denying the truth isolates me even more. Conversely, if they said they knew I was going to die, I would believe them and be terribly upset.

Some hesitate to touch on my health at all, oblivious, erasing discomfort, or fearful that they will remind me of something that I will never forget. Outside, looking in, they have no idea how deeply mired I am in my ills when they discount and move on. Diminishing pain does not dissipate it, denials and minimizations abandon me in it.

Others shy away from sharing any of their own hardships with me, or do so with a comparative and dismissive apology. I lovingly remind them that it's not a competition. Applying a hierarchy to pain and ranking suffering is a pointless contest, with no winners and no losers.

*   *   *

One needn't look far to see from whom my values were instilled. Self-sufficient and accomplished, I didn't build my prized strength of character and independence being mollycoddled by my adoring parents. I have no doubt that they both love me more than life itself, as I do them. They have served me generously with devotion, though their loyalties do know boundaries and their priorities escape me at times. Having well earned their respect, I no longer need their discipline and criticism. I crave their unabridged consideration and care, their protection, their empathy.

My father often proudly associates his drive with John F. Kennedy's inspiring speech. "We choose to go to the moon in this decade and do the other things, not because they are easy, but because they are hard, because that goal will serve to organize and measure the best of our energies and skills, because that challenge is one that we are willing to accept, one we are unwilling to postpone, and one which we intend to win." I respect his ambitious encouragement, but the last thing a highly functioning overachiever in crisis needs is a trip to the moon.

I could continue to multitask as a daddy's girl and as a self-standing woman, if only his intellectual push didn't so frequently come to shove. In response to the weakness I displayed when answering a polite question about how I was feeling, my empathetically impaired father pondered, wrote and delivered a *Why me, why not me?* manifesto, with inspirational intent. I regret my pathetic answer more than his insensitive reply.

I will not see my father come to terms with what befell his advantaged daughter. Though caring and emotional, he is protective in theory and tends to me from a safe distance, while my husband and mother step in without armor. Signs of distress or pessimism from my end are met with disapproval and disappointment from his end. Guilty of too many gifts, how dare I flounder amid my spoil of riches. Perhaps he operates from a place of fear-induced denial. He needs to see me exert my character and then he will know that I can still do anything, that I can survive. We are so close and committed, but sadly I feel the gap, let go, and perform for him as expected. He does not live in my world, nor does he understand it.

*   *   *

Usually willing to share, I have stock answers and guide conversations with redirections as I see fit, in both social and clinical settings. I quickly learn who truly wants and can handle the unvarnished truth, and who can't. I try not to distress the latter with what they don't want to hear.

Above all else, I preserve and protect my body and soul. I am justified, though under absolutely no obligation to justify. I owe no access nor explanation, physical and emotional boundaries are mine to define and enforce. Sensitive to whom I let in and under what terms, I guard my wellbeing and limited reserves of energy, with attention to cause and effect.

*   *   *

Once, I was nearly unflappable. Now, I am sensitive to innocent, encouraging comments. When grasping for a lifeline, there is absolutely no reassuring sense of choice or control.

Under catastrophic circumstances, minimizing and dismissive silver linings tarnish on delivery and are hardly comforting. Being handed a half-full glass is not helpful at all. It's a preposterous notion that deserves to be thrown against a wall, shattered. While my optimistic father will opine that I have nothing to drink from, my sympathetic husband will suggest that I drink from my shoe.

There is a fine line between sharing in my appreciation and reminding me of my good fortune, as if I'm unaware or undeserving. For everything I have been born into, gifted with and worked for, I live in a state of clarity and gratitude. Without disadvantages, I recognize that my vast personal and clinical resources are exemplary. Under different circumstances, this would surely have been a short obituary. With sincere empathy, it's no consolation that I don't live in a third world country and am not burdened with even more debilitating conditions. Blessed and cursed, fortunate and unfortunate, lucky and unlucky, I appreciate my privileges without guilt.

*   *   *

Exposed, I am left with little to harbor and to hold. Life just outside the inside comes with countless invisible and identifiable distressing intrusions. Cameras lay bare the most intimate and private moments of my incapacity, every image is transportive. Photographs from the year before will forever send a cold chill down my spine, when I look into my unknowing eyes. I resent requested or stolen snapshots, vehemently averse to the assault, insensitivity and gall. My state of recovery will always be in the foreground of images from the year after, no matter who flanks me or the landscape.

Various triggers add salt to my wounds. Tig Notaro's brilliant *One Mississippi* series is ripe with dark comedy, I enjoyed it despite the painful scene with her mother's last breaths. No one could anticipate when they recommended *My Octopus Teacher* that the documentary would lead me to associate with the main character and vividly imagine my own body wasting away, in full view, for all the world to see. Nor could the uninitiated pontificating belaboredly on death and world miseries during a dinner party imagine my overwhelming desire to evict them from our home to the cold curb.

With silence and a slow smile, I secretly deliver inappropriate commentary awards to my loved ones, and amuse myself with my snarky inner replies.

- "Will you have cosmetic surgery?" To revise the appearance of my abdominal scar, hell no.

- "I don't know how you do it. I would kill myself." How encouraging!

- "Other women are dealing with not being able to get to the salon to get their hair done (due to COVID shutdowns), at least you don't have to worry about that." Lucky me!

- "We can discuss a plant-based diet when you get through your trauma." Emaciated and reliant on protein, I could literally eat a horse.

- "The worst thing in the world is cold French fries." Seriously?!

*   *   *

Heartfelt awards would go to my oldest and newest friends. One so sympathetic to my pain that she genuinely wishes she could trade places with me, though I would never let her. One who will read this draft and ache to reach through the pages to hug me, to hold my hand, to scream on my behalf. My community is so abundant and generous in their ministries, I would need a truckload of medals to compensate every benevolent act…

An unexpected comrade is an emotional literacy poster child, reminding me that "it might turn out so...but not today." He acknowledges my trepidation, how highly discomfiting it is that we are not living in ordinary times, how the pandemic has induced an amplified sense of foreboding. He sagely writes "The captain of the Titanic was 'confident' his ship wouldn't sink and we know how that went. I do follow the maxim of the Sully Sullenbergers of the world…when the odds are long you only have two choices. I'll take the shot and go for broke. You have great medical resources, a resolute spirit and the profound support of your husband. Your dice keep rolling up right and just might stay that way even if it seems so damnably uncertain now." His eloquent words are balm to my soul and give me courage, bless him.

*   *   *

In *Please Send Hats*, Laura Clark-Hansen explores bragging rights and the concept of ultracrepidarianism–the habit of giving opinions and advice on matters outside of one's knowledge or competence. "Some people try to comfort cancer survivors by saying, 'We're all going to die. I could be hit by a bus tomorrow.'

Have you been running from the bus for years? Getting hit by the proverbial bus is not the same as being pursued by it, watching it gain on you as you approach each check-up, only to have it veer off at the last minute, leaving you breathless and choking on the sickening fumes of fear that it leaves behind. If you haven't literally been there, let me assure you that it isn't the same as worrying about the possibility of getting hit by a bus."

As a cancer survivor, you know in fact that the bus exists, that it is gunning for you, with a full tank of gas. You even know the year, the make, the model and the color. Statistics have mapped out when and where your paths may cross, and you have an exacting sense of the personal and collateral damage it will do. You know the driver and that he is actively seeking you out, you can see the whites of his eyes. On a good day, you can hear the engine, rumbling in the distance. On a bad day, the engine's roar obliterates all other sound. That bus is in hot pursuit!

*   *   *

Overzealous, I seize opportunities to make good use of my lessons. A fixer by nature, my tendency is to share and problem solve. I inspire, coach, mentor, direct and lead freely, even when I really shouldn't. I shudder to think of my countless all-knowing missteps… Of how many times I have presumed that I could relate to experiences or intuit another human being's feelings.

I have become more aware of language, how it is used and what it delivers. I'm irked when sincerity and experience are diminished with "honestly" and "I feel like," especially when communication is critical, and I attempt to strike the prefaces from my vocabulary.

*   *   *

In mayhem, there is a tendency to step in or away. Exuberant on the subject of birth, the average person falters when facing the subject of mortality, especially in the case of those who are not old nor long infirm. With a sigh of relief, few people hold their close position when they believe the dust has settled.

Perpetually distracted and electronically connected to the intangible, we are often unable to be wholly present with ourselves, let alone with others. More concerned about over-stepping than under-stepping, we sacrifice connectivity.

A compassionate response requires no special skills. Simply abandoning attempts to evade, analyze or control other's pain enables us to extend empathy and thereby lend a salve to the burn. When there is no question to answer or remedy to the hurt, we must simply learn to lock eyes and hold hands.

SHADES OF GRAY

June 2020

"Worry is like a rocking chair. It gives you something to do but never gets you anywhere."

Erma Bombeck

Long after my last infusion, chemotherapy lashings continue with a reign of lingering collateral damage. With careful tending, I thought my nails had escaped treatments unscathed. I am shocked and repulsed when I notice my toenail detaching. One by one, I witness my nails succumb to the trauma. Sensitive, with opaque white and angry black demarcations, they lift from their beds. My toenail falls off in a final and revolting act of surrender.

My plight is now in plain view. An ever-present reminder of lethal illnesses and lethal treatments, I am exposed in all my degradation. From my bald head and hairless body, to my atrophied muscles and sickened skin, to my scarred neck, abdomen and arms, to my disfigured torso, groin, ankle and foot, to my ruined finger and toenails. Pained and traumatized on the outside, I am discomfited and shamed on the inside. It's not just that I don't feel feminine, I don't feel human. There is little good left of me.

*   *   *

With my life in shambles, I am in bereavement for the past I treasured and the future I trusted. Seven months in, I still cannot shake my disbelief or digest our new reality. I live in the shadow of my former self, weak and clinging to remnants of my sanity. Brain-damaged by the duress of an exotic reality, my mental faculties have decayed, worn down and away. Wasted and frail, I am barraged by intrusive thoughts and have lost my peace of mind.

Freedom is lost to my incarceration, liberty does not exist in the confines of an incurable and deadly assignment. I will stay shackled to this disease for as long as I survive it. Calm, cool and collected no more, I cower in my wretched state under the heavy threat of my untimely demise.

*   *   *

My oncologist spoon feeds me. Just as I've swallowed my last bite, I am introduced to targeted maintenance drugs. I have been liberated from one toxic treatment regimen to be subjected to another. With the latest ghastly plan laid out, I will take a PARP inhibitor daily, for the rest of my life, or for as long as I can tolerate it. Literally, a small pill to swallow. Figuratively, a daily physical and psychological reminder that I must continue to fight back 24/7 to keep death at bay.

My disappointment is heart-wrenching. Always reliant, nothing I ever give or take is enough. It is impossible to divorce myself from the insidious disease that has sought so hard to claim me and still wants nothing more than to consume me. Gasping for air, I am unable to swim to the surface. I cannot breathe. There will be no return to the life I had.

*   *   *

Equally horrified by the effects of taking the drug and the risks of not taking it, I cannot refute the opportunity for a better outcome.

Safe handling instructions are alarming, no one should lay bare hands on the remedy that I must conceive to ingest. My Medal-of-Honor deserving husband will spare me over the course of my treatment. He will manage insurance and supplemental coverage, coordinate refills, delivery schedules and signatures with the specialty pharmacy and transit companies, store the vial out of my sight and set dosage reminders that he follows without a single miss. At home, in transit and abroad, he will leave a capsule by my pasted toothbrush every evening without fail. I am left with only one task, though more times than not my throat closes in resistance, and I must force myself to swallow.

*   *   *

The drug is not benign. My ambitious goal is to establish base line wellness with an acceptable level of toxicity. Ideally, it will stave off recurrence of the cancer I have had or have, without causing an ancillary cancer or other debilitating or deadly condition.

Off to a poor start, my absolute neutrophils nearly bottom out, leaving my already severely compromised immune system catastrophically crippled. With my life in jeopardy, there is talk of a bone marrow transplant. On again, off again, weekly adjustments and tests eventually result in a dosage that I am able to tolerate, though not without significant effect.

Along with other nuisances, I will experience persistent joint aches and pains and shortness of breath during my course of treatment. My team of specialists grows even more impressive as I add a rheumatologist, pulmonologist and cardiologist to my expansive collection.

*   *   *

Contemplating the risk and reward, my trusted nurse asks if I'm willing to play the odds. Her greatest fear for me is cancer and I know that, heartfelt, she wants me to continue treatment.

With a lifeline and an anchor, I am tethered at both ends. And how quickly I will come to rely on this barbed gift, as I imagine the cancer simmering, one capsule away from boiling over in an explosive volcanic eruption. Pompeii too was once thriving and sophisticated, until it was claimed by Mount Vesuvius in 79 AD. Surviving is sucking the life out of me. My nerves are worn, forever frayed. I am exhausted in body and spirit, in perpetual motion, fighting and flying. I trust my nurse, follow her recommendation to carry on with treatment, and release my clinical concerns to her care. Tired and vacant, I disconnect.

*   *   *

I mistake new assignments as betrayals, not understanding that my oncologist isn't being evasive. She knows that my threshold for physical pain and emotional angst has been spent, replenished only by adrenaline to carry me through surgery, chemotherapy, maintenance therapy and all the ills before, during, and after. She spares and saves me with her every deliberate action and can only present me with the next task if I have endured the last. If I am still fit to stand, to step into my next stage of survival.

Had I known, had it all been laid out like I wanted, the magnitude of my conditions would have been too far beyond my comprehension to digest. Blinded by foresight, how easily I could have given up. Hopelessly lost and not wanting to fight a losing battle, yet inherently torn, still so very desperate to live.

*   *   *

My life is no longer black and white, and I falter in shades of gray. A far cry from the polished, controlled and icy under pressure me of old, I am now prone to breakdowns and bouts of hysteria. Alternately numb and in excruciating pain, my physical and mental health is an Escher-esque elevator. I ride up and down, down and up, motion sick in minute-by-minute cycles. Presuming that I can pick up and move on, that each step forward is secure on an upward path, I am astonished and dismayed to stumble into crevice after crevice.

When my counselor asks if I can imagine feeling vulnerable without panicking, I laugh heartily and holler "Hell no!" My new guru, Brené Brown, describes "having the courage to show up when you can't control the outcome…courage does not exist without vulnerability." All this time, I mistook being brave and daring for being courageous, not realizing the powerful asset seated deep inside me.

*   *   *

My professional and personal resources are ceaseless in their care and encouragement, lending a hand when my strength and spirits wane. I am down in a ditch, not depressed in a well with sides that cannot be scaled. I counter my falls with determination to rise to the occasion, to define myself by the life I live. Striving to stay inspired, when my reserves run dry, I try again for my loved ones, if not for myself.

Continuing to play empowering word games, I seek:

Calm in Panic

Confidence in Fear

Faith in Despair

Order in Lack of Control

Security in Insecurity

Strength in Weakness

Healing in Pain

Gains in Losses

Joy in Devastation

Tranquility in Desperation

Hope in Hopelessness

Success in Defeat

*   *   *

Defensive and in denial, I am offended by accusations of anxiety and stoically unwilling to subject myself to symptomatic treatment with pharmaceuticals. In the 1980s, psychologist James Prochaska developed a transtheoretical model of behavior change with stages: pre-contemplation, contemplation, preparation, action and maintenance. Today's consumers desire a quick fix, and it's much easier to swallow a pill than to do the heavy lifting of looking inside yourself.

Guided by my counselor, the responsibility for actioning change lies squarely on my shoulders, and I tend to my situational anxiety the old-fashioned way, with loads of hard work over the long course of my cancer journey.

*　　　　　*　　　　　*

Grandmothers are generally excellent sources of knowledge and my counselor's is no exception. Her spirit reminds me not to poison the present with borrowed or wasted worry, with defeatist thinking. I charge myself to not squander good days with bad thoughts. A more optimistic approach will cost me nothing and have infinite returns. Emulating my husband, I imagine survival and consider futures that bring me joy.

To get there is a challenge that requires the intervention of my own paternal grandmother. Too well-behaved with her to ever warrant the action, I remember her touting the sure-fire remedy to a child's temper tantrum being a splash of cold water to the face. She may or may not have known that this triggers the mammalian diving reflex, a survival response that slows the heart rate and activates the parasympathetic nervous system.

In fight or flight mode, it can be impossible to think clearly. When our nervous system is operating in overdrive and so overwhelmed that all we can do is lash out or shut down, it becomes flooded and requires a reset. When hot and bothered, cold water can literally put out our internal fires. With a relentless need to escape a moment that never ends, the answer may be as simple as H_2O!

*　　　　　*　　　　　*

My emotional advances are even more onerous than my physical healing. One-dimensional intellectual investments limit my growth, I gain footing in every experience without a tragic ending. Anxiety accompanies each trial and tribulation, though reminders of the many times I haven't been doomed lend a valuable lesson. Step by step, my confidence increases through action and practice. I build endurance, find stability, and have yet to end up in a lifeless heap at the bottom of a staircase. Manic highs and lows will slowly equalize with each passing experience. I will lie low to weather the storms, with facts under my belt.

I shape acceptance with awareness, using a perspective scale to compartmentalize discomfort into a navigable timeframe.
- Five seconds or minutes are a non-issue, to be discounted.
- Five hours or days is a minor issue, to be quantified.
- Five weeks or months is an issue worthy of my time and attention.

*   *   *

Always the impatient overachiever seeking success, my finger is constantly on the pulse of my progress. I monitor how I am faring and lament my ongoing struggles, my incremental healing.

Frustrated when failing to thrive and asking my counselor to revisit the same issues, I realize that the solutions are all in my well stocked arsenal. There are not singular potions for dealing with diagnosis related anxiety, versus testing anxiety, versus anxiety about the insecurity of my future. I am reminded that toxic perfectionism is self-abuse of the highest order and to reset my expectations to a more realistic level.

*   *   *

While I will fail to exorcise anxiety in its entirety, I learn to contain it. I know that it has no positive value and recognize it for what it is and isn't. Anxiety is a cruel dramatist, a liar, Chicken Little. It is untrustworthy, harmful, toxic to mind and body, corrosive, abusive and a pessimistic sadist. It is physical and emotional distress and suffering. Misleading, it does not problem solve, nor is it predictive. Its nature is purely destructive and addictive.

I have been trained to watch for signs and triggers, a darkening mood, detachment, evening. To recognize what is real versus perceived. To redirect and apply solutions. I counter anxious thoughts with three better but believable alternatives. I use my well-honed management skills to identify and re-assign it, handle it the same way I would other unsolvable issues. I don't take the bait, I disassociate and let it be. Instead of distressing over the unchangeable past or unknowable future, I choose to empower myself in the now.

*   *   *

According to all my practitioners, a walk outside continues to be the most healing balm for body and soul. One step in front of the other, we are built for movement…forward.

When I am not holding my breath, huffing, puffing and dramatically sighing, I try not to waste air. I endeavor to give my body the oxygen it wants and needs.

My carefully scripted mission statement to preserve inner tranquility is hit or miss…
- Do not allow inner voices/images to run riot.
- Pause/interrupt with authority to disempower the cycle/self-abuse.
- Actively choose to accept or discount thoughts with ownership.
- Anchor and redirect to a pathway towards peace.
- Choose to be present, to relax, reassure yourself.
- Inhale calm… Exhale chaos…

*   *   *

According to Buddha, "The secret of health for mind and body is not to mourn for the past, it is not to worry about the future, it is not to anticipate troubles, it is simply to live in the present moment wisely and earnestly."

Swinging wildly from pessimistic to optimistic extremes, I labor my way back to realism. I learn to be careful with seemingly benign words, I know their inspirational powers to give or take away. *If* does not mean *when*, and hypothetical speculation is the enemy of calm.

Inaction is hard for me, though I learn to recognize when I need to be still. I strive to release my "make it happen" mentality, to live between the I must do everything and I can do nothing.

*   *   *

Violently shoved into the unknown, I now know what I am made of. Against all science and sense, there are times that the human spirit rises, more powerful than anything in its path.

RITES OF PASSAGE

July 2020

"We cannot direct the wind, but we can adjust our sails."
Bertha Calloway

The ruby is a prized and powerful stone, long considered to yield good fortune to the body, mind and soul. Ancient warriors in Burma and China adorned their armor with the gem to provide protection in battle. Believing it promised invincibility, some even went so far as to insert the gems into their own flesh.

During my second hospital stay, a cafeteria worker interacted with my husband daily, asking after me, praying for me, and gifting me with a bracelet she made. Named for my birthstone, I never laid eyes on her yet know her by heart.

*   *   *

Aesthetically passionate, I clean house and ruthlessly obliterate sickness souvenirs. There will be no clinical documents, drugs, medical devices, physical therapy bands, wigs or headcovers lying about. Out of sight, they are only out of mind until revealed in a closet or drawer–ever present reminders and promises that they are there for me, should I need them again. In daring and cathartic acts, I will purge items when they are no longer of use. I brave tempting fate by letting go of those hateful hooks, deeply embedded into an atrocious past and a future I hope to avoid.

I spare only the personal cards and letters I have received. Eventually, I will release those too and free an antique Asian box from its oppressive weight. When I look at the box now, it is no longer a red coffin. The porcupine quill that I discovered along an abandoned Roman aqueduct in Umbria secures the lock to liberty. It is light with beauty.

*   *   *

Zodiac signs reportedly originated with Babylonian astronomy during the first millennium BC. While I do not rely on astrology, I find it vaguely curious, especially since I can now associate both my arrival and possibly preordained departure from this planet in my given sign.

Though I would much prefer to be a Leo, I was born a Cancer. The brave crab was sent to this earth both unaware of its strength and a fiercely protective fighter when motivated. By nature, Cancers are tenacious, highly imaginative, sympathetic, persuasive and impatient. Caring, loving and kind, we are faithful and loyal for as long as we feel safe and satisfied.

My husband does not believe in astrology at all, though was nonetheless born a Pisces. As two Water signs, Cancer and Pisces connect through emotions, usually as soon as they lay eyes on each other. Brought together by romantic love, we nurture and cherish one another with pleasure.

*   *   *

Livid, frustrated and fit to be tied, I cannot escape my demons. This is absurd, outrageous, a condemnation for my sinful unions. Who could imagine that I would be the one reliant on care when I should be the caregiver. I terrorize myself imagining something happening to my husband, imagining our mutual incapacitation. Crippling fears before are paralyzing fears now. I will remain permanently unnerved at the most benign signs of his aging or mortality.

Forgoing my independence to receive his ministries, he actively participates in my healing process without lording it over me. He proudly manages all the mechanics of my maintenance and spares me from mundane tasks. He is my adept agent, my dealer and distributor, my everything. Without an ounce of energy to spare,

I love his physical and emotional care and hate my dependence and reliance on it.

Nearly always aligned, we are equals in our determination and grit when our tempers rarely flare. Only once do I rail awfully and in a tantrum tell him to go, to cut his losses…as if I can live without him.

When he calls me Beautiful, an old term of endearment, it feels like a lie. A reference to what was, not what is. I fear that he will remember the horrors over the highlights, that seeing me so debilitated has spoiled his view of me. That I have failed in my intentions and promises, that I have ruined the rest of his life.

*   *   *

Having taken my longevity for granted, I am now hyperaware of my mortality. Facing deadly diagnoses, the risk of imminent death before, during and immediately after my hospitalizations and during treatment has enlightened me. I may or may not purge this vile, odious thief.

My oncologist monitors my numerous conditions. All hands are on deck to make me well. Lymphedema treatments progress from intensive wrappings and therapy with yet another specialized practitioner to the conceptual freedom of a strangling compression stocking that I am unable to put on or take off without assistance. My first mammogram is executed, I imagine the inventor having his testicles pressed between a dictionary and bible by a pedantic zealot. Monthly labs, quarterly CA125, abdominal and chest CTs and pelvic exams, and an order for a colonoscopy add layers of dread to my to-do list.

Channeling Winston Churchill, I keep going through my hell and realize my forty-seventh birthday after all. Ever the planner, I adjust my lifeline and anticipate that I will not survive my fiftieth birthday. If I do, I will surely not make it through that year and will meet my end within a tidy half-century marker.

*   *   *

I live bridging the gap of my narrow escape, closer to the end and in mourning with countless quiet goodbyes. I lay in wait, filled with terror at the images of my life prior and my loved ones' lives after.

Egotistical and possessive, I cannot imagine my life without them, nor, worse yet, can I imagine their lives without me. My parents cannot be made to suffer my abandonment, I cannot stomach the thought of neglecting them, nor can I stomach the thought of them neglecting me. Deeply committed, I can only bear envisioning my husband's future nurtured with my adoring care. Others in my sphere may mourn me, marked, not marred, by my absence.

When my fire is extinguished, life will go on. Every dawn will distance those I have left in my wake from the loss. New people and experiences will take my place. The memory of me will matter less with each passing day.

Vanishing in both body and spirit, I will eventually cease to exist in my entirety, and I'm not happy about it. Historically, my "I'm not happy!" declarations demand prompt attention, I act or spur action elsewhere to be made happy. In this case though, there is little to do.

*   *   *

I admire, though cannot absorb, other cultures that both address and embrace death as a natural process, celebrating the end with equal vigor to the beginning. Ironically, last summer I read *Reimagining Death: Stories and Practical Wisdom for Home Funerals and Green Burials* by Lucina Herring, while simultaneously reading *Midwest Foraging* by Lisa Rose. My family was alarmed and questioned anything ingestible that I prepared or served during that time. The film *Departures* delicately captures the honorous Japanese encoffinment ceremony. The naturally decomposing bodies in Sally Mann's *Hold Still: A Memoir with Photographs* both repulsed and fascinated me.

In The Game of Things, my last words are "I'm madder than hell and not going to take it anymore." To peals of laughter, I give away my answer and cry happily because it's funny and true. More stirring responses include "A life well lived."

*   *   *

I share an epiphany with my counselor, our fixer. My ongoing emotional struggles with recurrence are rooted in my impatient nature. If I'm dying, or going to die, I'd just as soon get it over with. The suspense is killing me!

*   *   *

In *Being Mortal: Medicine and What Matters in the End*, Atul Gawande writes "Death is the enemy. But the enemy has superior forces. Eventually, it wins. And in a war that you cannot win, you don't want a general who fights to the point of total annihilation. …the damage is greatest if all you do is battle to the bitter end."

I am vehemently opposed to clinging to life at all cost, yet equally opposed to dying. Visions of recurrence and means to a torturous end are inescapable. Backed into a corner and trapped, my burden is too heavy to live with and too real to evade. I am in the sickening position of defending my freedom and future by imagining the delivery of a fatal blow.

The one thing that I will not abide by is a bird's eye view to my extended degradation. I refuse to wither away under assessment, with an audience tracking all the little losses of life that occur as my body fails me in the most cruel and inhumane ways.

In *Memoir of a Debulked Woman: Enduring Ovarian Cancer*, Susan Gubar writes "A person with cancer dies in increments, and a part of you slowly dies with them. Disease may score a direct hit on only one member of a family, but shrapnel tears the flesh of the others. Life at any price does not seem a meaningful goal… Who does not entertain the flickering impulse to snip life hanging by a thread?"

*   *   *

Lurking behind the polished surface of control is a rich, omnipotent imagination. Because I suffer from detailed and reeling thoughts, I find comfort in openly addressing my worries. I ponder how I can protect myself, skirt a life of pointless suffering and dependency.

Fatalism is weak with inaction, I learn to live in fear by confronting it. I won't be caught off guard again, in a perpetual state of blindly stumbling forward, following a prescribed plan that I haven't had any part in, led again by the hands of strangers. Blind to my future, my existence is within my power. As much care as I've put into curating our life, how could I not want to orchestrate the end with dignity?

*   *   *

Perhaps I can quiet my ruminations with a well devised plan. With self-discipline, I ground and empower myself, gain a sense of my lost control. Systematically annihilate inadequacies and move forward with perfect resets, instructions and timelines via streamlined routes. Bridging the gulf between my ideals and reality, I spin garbage into gold.

When the life I have isn't enough of a life to sustain, I will make my last act of impatience one to hurry nature along its course. I don't actively seek knowledge but do pay rapt attention to what drugs combined with alcohol will peacefully still a beating heart.

With a final courageous act, my people and I will be spared from futile care, though they may argue that they were robbed of time and an opportunity to say goodbye. My husband especially, not because I don't love him enough, because I love him too much. With one exception, I intend to gift them and myself with a preserved memory, sans the wrenching drama of my final breath.

*   *   *

My mother will have the heart and backbone to honor me. I am aware of how she watches me, stands sentry, observing everything. I feel her scrutiny, her worry. She takes it all in, aware, protective and resigned. She misses nothing.

A realist, like her daughter, her vision is clear, unobscured by the blurring and blunting forces of the emotionally unimaginable. She both venerates and shames me, with responsibility and admonishments for mismanaging my health, because I should have known better than the oblivious masses.

Grounded in truth, she sees me, and I know that she alone could endure my last selfish and brazen request. An inconceivable final maternal castigation, should I ask her to inflict it. Her ceaseless love, compassion and dedication will yield salvation, in my first and last breaths.

*   *   *

I set the stage, on a bender to make my mark and leave an optimally ordered world. Our nest is handsomely feathered and I further my imprint with monograms. In my sight line, there are orchids and violets–plants, life. I wonder if my husband will take care of them, if he will maintain his own wellness–drink enough water, eat well, exercise, be saintly without me. My addled mind is made more miserable pondering each of the million unanswered and unanswerable questions that I continue to conjure.

Operating from wells of desire and pits of despair, I organize a detailed plan for my celebration of life, including venue, menu, music and pictures. I hope that my organs will be salvageable and repurposed, however anticipate that the cancer will also eradicate my ability to make my body of use to others. I stop just short of writing my own obituary, though I intend to do that too. I have every intention of maintaining control from the grave, yet I don't want to be buried, or burned, or anything other than alive and well.

*　　　　*　　　　*

Patrick Henry said "Give me liberty or give me death!" and I agree, in principle. On the other hand, I know life in captivity intimately, and it ain't all bad. I may never cross paths with cancer again. I may know or never know recurrence, acquiesce to or deny treatment plans, gain something or lose everything, though I am unlikely to live through the end of time. I ground my fears of the unknown in the knowledge that, while I can't choose the mortal battles that may befall me, I can choose to fight or surrender. Life is mine to live or leave.

Well prepared for the outcome I most fear and expect, I liberate myself to imagine the outcome I most desire. My vision reaches far into the future, into the hours before any horrific disease should befall my husband or recur to me... Preserving our precious unity, I envision us many moons from now on a spectacular adventure, perhaps painlessly slipping into a crevice in the pristine Italian Alps to take our last breath together. Wrapped in each other's arms in death as we were in life–healthy, happy and whole. Intertwined in body and spirit, always. Going out on a high note, with flair, together, doing what we loved. Our beautiful lives conserved, saved. Our memory for others romantic, poetic even.

*　　　　*　　　　*

Nearly 2,000 years ago, Epictetus, a venerable philosopher born enslaved in the eastern outreaches of the Roman Empire, established these guiding principles:

Know what you can control and what you can't.
Harmonize your actions with the way life is.
Accept events as they occur.
Your will is always within your power.
Make full use of what happens to you.
Act well the part that is given to you.
Conduct yourself with dignity.
Stay the course, in good weather and bad.
Caretake this moment.

This ancient text grounds and guides me, it is my newly adopted religion. What I look for is what I will see, and I am tasked with staying in my lane.

TRUTH AND DARE

August 2020

"Take the gentle path."

George Herbert

My body is recognizable to the casual observer, only I know the depths of my damages. In less than a year I've gone from my most powerful self to my most pitiful self, not yet realizing that surviving is the most powerful act of all.

I catch glimpses of myself that I recognize. In the soft morning light, I look down on my lithe body, the shadows obscure the scars. In these moments, I forget, displace recent events for an instant, comforted by a glance or touch at what I knew to be lost.

With the slightest shift, shocking backlash effects bridge the distance that I have travelled in the millisecond it takes to interpret the mutilations I see marring my flesh. Reeled back to reality, I am reminded of everything all at once, then go back and pretend, steal one more minute.

The Japanese art of kintsugi involves repairing broken objects with gold. The flaw is seen as a unique piece of the object's history, which adds to its beauty. A thing is beautiful not in spite of the damage it suffered but because of the damage. In a less pained future, I will look up to my body, in awe and admiration.

*　　　　　*　　　　　*

My physical therapist, husband and I make a dream team and have achieved a monumental win. Anticipating the support of a knee brace and cane through the end of the year while my femoral nerve labors to repair itself, my recently wasted muscles have never been more toned, defined and responsive. Following our series of Olympian feats, my therapist releases me from her skilled care with longstanding homework assignments. Praise her, praise him and praise me, I have been healed!

As overjoyed as I am with the accomplishment and my newfound liberty, her release is bittersweet. I have become dependent on her guidance and am most secure under the care of her keen mind and perceptive hands.

My treasured therapist is an architect and rebuilds me, she is the sole body practitioner who does me no harm. Of all my clinicians, she knows my body best and will continue to serve me when I am in need over the course of many years. Beyond femoral nerve therapy, abdominal and pelvic floor rehabilitation will address scarring, adhesions, protrusions, undulations, pain and paranoia. I take solace in her knowledge and gentle touch.

*   *   *

Like Mrs. Potato Head, I patch myself together with faux lashes and a remarkably realistic acrylic toenail, toxic glue be damned. My hair slowly grows back, and I am born again. From the first irregular shadows of growth, it will be nearly one year post-treatment until I have just enough to tangle my fingers in. Childlike, I obsessively self-soothe, stroking my scalp and twirling my tufts. I will reemerge in the guises of G.I. Jane, a shorn poodle, Don King, Rod Stewart and Tina Turner circa 1993. Wild curls yield gnarly knots, morph into dreadlocks, and in two years to less interesting, more familiar tresses. My fingernails will grow back as well, though short bedded and with lasting sensitivity.

*   *   *

The average human hair is only 70 microns thick. From the madness of its loss to the elation of its growth, it proves to be one of my most trying and impactful life lessons.

Tentative and emboldened, my first outings without a headcover are epic. A regular at medical centers, the staff are welcoming and easily identify me in all my iterations and disguises. In the general public, I cause confusion because my appearance is constantly changing. Some people don't recognize me, repeatedly, and I become adept at reintroducing myself. A dear friend is enthused during her first sighting and asks to pet me, I happily accept her tender loving touch. When an unknowing acquaintance sees me, he stills the room when he loudly exclaims "What did you do to your hair?!" I ease the poor dear with my "You don't want to know…" reply and a warm smile. Apologetic gentleman aside, I will receive more sincere compliments on head coverings and my shorn and growing hair than I have in over four decades left to my own coiffure devices.

*   *   *

Downfalls breed curiosity and the wind is sucked from my sails when those in the know ask if I plan to keep my hair short or if I will let it grow. The bristling questions intimate control, yet my choice was life or death. Extremely tentative of assuming ownership of my future, I lack the bandwidth to expose myself to unchartered territory. Insecure and precariously hanging on to my new role, I have been nurturing regrowth by the millimeter and brainwashing myself to live in the now. It's easier for me to imagine losing my hair again to the ravages of another round of chemotherapy than to imagine the two or three years it will take to feel it skim the base of my scarred neck, or sweep across my clavicle.

During one of my early militaristic outings, I receive a compliment from a stranger who says she wishes she was brave enough for such a short cut. Given a chance to rise above my past traumas, I don't squander the opportunity by pointlessly opening a wound, or drag an innocent stranger down with me. Embracing her positivity, I choose not to define myself by a disease, and thereby minimize its impact on our lives. As much control as I may lack, when my wits are about me, I am determined to select power over pity every time. I thank her and encourage her to go for it. In that moment, I don't feel like a victim. I feel like a million dollars!

*   *   *

Fastidious and meticulous before, for the next year, a single strand of hair will harshly remind me of my losses when least expected. My knowing and protective husband eventually tells me that he has been intercepting and disposing of American Cancer Society accoutrement catalogs when he collects the mail, immediately dispatching the reminder to our recycling bin. He only mentions this in passing, to inform me that he finally called to ask them to remove my name and address from their distribution list.

Three years later, I will still acutely respond to triggers. When I pass a pharmacy window in Bergen, Norway and a display of head coverings causes me to catch my breath, I say nothing though my husband and I hold hands and he likely feels my grip tighten. A tsunami of emotions well to my surface. I inhale, exhale, measure now versus then, swallow my angst, and I move forward.

*   *   *

The human body is biologically and culturally built for adaptation, and though I may never find tranquility, biological plasticity dictates that I will find a way to live well within the bounds of my constraints. Accustomed to flourishing in my before and fractured in body and mind in my now, my irretrievably lost confidence can only be built anew. It will be a different existence than what I had known, but it will be a meaningful, informed and honest existence.

I learn to adjust to life in a constant state of heightened alarm, to dull my response mechanisms to real and perceived threats, to live with vulnerability. I assuage my regrets and fears, aim to accept external events as they occur, and consider how I want to carry on. I continue to step away from panic and anxiety, work my way through consternation to resilience. I envision my peaceful body and confident mind being anchored on solid ground and I rally, one square inch at a time.

*   *   *

Psychologist and Researcher Ron Siegel separates two arrows from a Buddhist lesson. Life shoots the first arrow when something difficult happens. The first arrow invites us to develop a fierce inner nurturer, who stands opposite the inner critic, to witness and tend to the pain, to find a salve for the initial injury. We shoot the second arrow, when we add to our pain and suffering by how we talk to ourselves and others about what is happening with us.

In refusing to allow inner dialogue to contribute to our injuries and in comforting ourselves, we may transcend the boundaries of when our pain began or when it will end. At opposite ends, dread and hope are rooted in our imagination. The choice is into which pool we will dip our quill.

OUTRAGEOUS FORTUNE

September 2020

"Flectere si nequeo superos, acheronta movebo."
(If I cannot reach heaven, I will raise hell.)

Virgil

My own personal Armageddon has led me to life in limbus, the region on the border of hell. With no promise of a cure, my wellness is in constant question and I am apprehensive day and night. Teetering uncertainly on that edge, recurrence menacingly nips at my heels. I actively consider, dismiss and report from a narrow surveillance ledge. It is no more than one foot wide and I'm spent waiting, anticipating when it will all come crashing down again, vividly imagining how. Hungry for insight, my fractured toes grip the rim as I lean in towards the unknown. My muscles are tense as I strain forward to peer into the depths of the abyss, where there is nothing to see.

Just as I contemplate diving in to meet my ender, I realize that I am also at risk of losing my balance and step back. Unchecked hypervigilance will consume the life that I'm supposed to be living, yielding fear as my constant companion. I can afford myself another ninety-nine feet and the ground is right there, waiting for me. I can spare myself life on the precipice, there is comfort to be had in purgatory.

*   *   *

My second post-treatment CTs miraculously bear no evidence of disease. With baited breath, I have survived the most critical recurrence period. My oncologist celebrates my milestone by telling me that she's done her part, that it's now up to me. In that moment, she releases her grip and ceases to hold my hand.

Referencing mountains and tracking my climb and position, she reports that I have gotten to the other side, that the struggle is behind me, though it isn't. My periods of rest are not unencumbered, I am under threat and tasked with a suspicious mind.

Both an honor and a burden, survivorship care plans will loom large over the course of five years, if I am lucky. The pleasure of anticipation has been displaced by the agony of measuring life by medical milestones. Life has become a series of intermissions in an endless opera, the drama is oppressive.

*   *   *

From the comfort of luxurious trappings, I live on pins and needles, constantly calculating risks and tracking how many lives I have left. Oblivious before and charged with knowing now, understanding, monitoring and assessing my health is a daunting assignment. Even more so when my nurse advises that most recurrences are identified by the patient, with symptoms mirroring their original vague presentations. With all senses heightened, in a state of constant scrutiny, I watch and wait for signs of my imminent demise.

When I graduate to longer reprieves between testing, my progress is marred by the paranoia of cells lying dormant, hibernating until a trigger is pulled. Every day that passes is one day further away from what happened, yet one day closer to what will happen next. My best hope is distance from both.

Amid celebratory dates and results, I am both relieved and depressed. My loved ones are impotent to free me of my burden, rather our shared burden. I reassure them when I can see straight, though they seem to believe what I never will. Stalked by a killer, my hackles are permanently raised.

*   *   *

Perpetually astonished by my medical history and vast array of specialists, routine exams are forever changed. In what will be a lasting physiological response in medical facilities, my heart races and blood pressure rises when my vitals are charted. Vulnerable and tense, despite mindful breathing practices, I draw in and expel embarrassingly ragged breaths on command.

Every appointment is now fraught with underlying tension. For over four decades, I was highly confident in my health. A lifetime of prior assumptions has vanished in mere months, leaving me petrified of what lurks beneath my surface. Absurd scenarios have become my new reality. I anticipate failure and brace myself for bad news. My only certainty is uncertainty.

*   *   *

Questionnaires and forms are hateful reminders of what was, and what still is. I chart my atrocious histological events and my chronic issues. Trying to find the right answers, selections are not always definitive, leaving cancer open-ended. I ponder surveillance status terminology–not curable, durable remission, disease free, no evidence of disease. It all sounds so temporary, so non-committal. Do I discount one for the other and magically welcome disease by declaring I do or don't have it, or did have it, or may again have it? I make my mark where I see fit and consciously move on to the next step, accepting that a history with cancer does not automatically translate into my present and future.

While human beings have yet to establish an infinite survivorship trajectory, at what point can I consider myself a survivor? At what point will I? Technically, following a cancer diagnosis, as long as you have a pulse you are a survivor.

*   *   *

I rein in terror in advance of every cancer screening, familiar testing routines and dread are my new dictates.

I anticipate the fasting, drive to the hospital, entry and arrival to outpatient testing, and the labs that precede the CTs. Among various gory fixations, plasma is one of my favored recurrent themes. My life under a microscope is charted hundreds of times, with six common lab orders that comprise forty-nine values. I borrow and waste worry left and right, pondering blood draws and how many gallons have been extracted from my veins.

I anticipate the CT preparations, the IV puncturing my skin and my inability to desensitize. My hour-long sipping and swallowing of contrast fluid, now a vile flavored shake full of artificial ingredients and sweeteners detrimental to my health. The technician, room and equipment. Automatically assuming the position on the table under the ornamental light panel, closing my eyes, and awaiting mechanical breathing instructions, directing me to inhale, hold and exhale…granting me permission to breathe normally. I anticipate the contrast coursing through my vascular system, the metallic pulse in my throat and the flood of heat in my groin. A second round of breathing on command. Exposure to yet another round of ionizing radiation, which is itself known to increase the risk of cancer. My escorted walk back to the lobby and reunion with my darling husband, who once nibbled on a chocolate chip cookie and sipped sparkling water from France to sustain himself while I was being scanned for signs that would seal our fate. While he calmly finishes his bottle of *Perrier*, I will drink a gallon of water to rid my body of the contrast agents and await results, certain that I have succumbed to the brutal end that befalls the vast majority of women with my condition.

In a viciously repetitive cycle with no end in sight, the relief of one result is quickly displaced by the apprehension of the next evaluation. I am inevitably immediately symptomatic and must remind myself that I just cleared testing, there could not possibly be disease advanced enough to present symptoms within the week following my CTs. The physical and emotional strain of confronting my mortality takes another wearing toll.

*   *   *

In *Memoir of a Debulked Woman: Enduring Ovarian Cancer,* Susan Gubar writes about cancer being a paranoia's dream come true. "There's something in there that I cannot see or feel or imagine, trying to murder me." While now aware of the barely discernable signs, my body is wrecked from the byproducts of cancer treatments and trying to heal itself. Even at its peak, the body's core mechanics never cease action. They are always and alarmingly in motion as I study my systems analytically from all angles. I waste so much time fast-forwarding to the end, desperate for unattainable certainty, whatever it may be.

Let down by everything I have done right, I stress about the stress that will encourage my damaged immune system to allow cells to turn on me again. With far more ease in my compromised body, surely and with savage determination they march along, preparing to divide and conquer, gearing up for round two.

*   *   *

I will wholeheartedly believe and emphatically declare that I am dying in various detailed iterations, ad infinitum. Twice, throbbing abdominal pains waken me, the Grim Reaper must be near. Changing positions, tea and a heating pad save me. After my second salvation, I consider the benign possibility that a BBQ dinner had simply caused digestive distress. A poor night disrupted by a migraine and nausea is certain to end badly. The migraines that I have suffered since adolescence are now chronic, signaling metastasis and brain tumors. After another narrow miss, I track back to my alcohol consumption the evening prior and decide to pare back. Foggy sensations in my chest and a dry unproductive cough are clear signs that my lungs are full of cancer. A random heart ache in the afternoon and evening promises a trip to the morgue. Lower back pain, bladder pressure and a full belly are all sure signs that my abdominal cavity is again under siege.

Three pounds lost or gained nag at my delicate psyche. Despite my generally organic whole-food diet, I find even natural carbohydrates, fruits, vegetables and plain yogurt threatening. Sugar is the devil–cancer loves it, and every granule is sure to feed its voracious cells. I believe that a single cookie could do me in, that a Tic Tac could be the final nail in my coffin.

General feelings of malaise indicate that my time is indeed coming to a close. Any discomfort at all is proof positive that I am being consumed from the inside out and on the verge of passing out of the picture. Every twinge, ache or pain that I would have once easily dismissed leads me straight to my grave as I imagine disease running rampant and my immediate spontaneous combustion.

*   *   *

Though my dramatic elucidations are always believable, they are rarely accurate. Despite my ambitious assumptions, my job is not to interpret symptoms, diagnose or define treatment plans (allegedly, I'm not qualified). As skilled as I am at anticipating threats and outcomes, my powers are limited. I can continue to torture myself or learn how to bear my doubts, suffer more skillfully, and charge myself with a burden of proof.

My people know that I am feral and they cannot control me, but they don't hesitate to rein me in when I run wild. There are no snake oil curses or cures. Case in point–when I am presented with converse scenarios (a person with a terrible diet eats one carrot and believes it to be curative), I see the absurdity of my ways. I made healthy choices before, and look what happened. I'm not going to succumb to this disease because I licked an ice cream cone or drank another glass of wine.

My teams guide me and I follow their self-care recommendations. I help myself and I also measure my quality of life. I don't go on benders, nor do I deprive myself of small pleasures. I hold on to my concerns but release my paranoia to Tajimamori, the god of sweets. If so inclined, I eat the cake!

*   *   *

In *TED Talk: What Almost Dying Taught Me About Living,* Suleika Jaouad states "You can be held hostage by the worst thing that's ever happened to you and allow it to hijack your remaining days, or you can find a way forward. It is far more radical and dangerous to have hope than to live hemmed in by fear."

Through extensive guidance and constant redirection, appropriate observation habits form and take shape. With the utmost expertise in my own body and health, I am to monitor myself from a safe distance. My challenge is to pay attention, to proficiently collect and report data. I endeavor to stay body focused while disengaging mentally, to believe evidence and to release judgment.

A historically high achiever, I now strive for and celebrate the unremarkable. There will be no partial relapse, the only 100% certainty is that there will be a recurrence or none at all.

*   *   *

I vacillate from soaring in survival to sinking back into helpless and hopeless despair, though spend more time alight than burning my feet in the fires of my hell. I will spend hours terrorizing myself by imagining and anticipating every possible threat and dire outcome, without conquering my fears or gaining peace of mind. The dynamic and motivating Brené Brown sparks emotional resilience in me, illuminating that "we can choose joy or to dress rehearse tragedy." If only I weren't so well adept at engaging in both, simultaneously.

In a crisis of biblical proportions, I seek clarity and calm. My logical mind takes hold, methodical, practical. I solve my solvable problems, aware of influence versus control, owning one and dismissing the other. I abandon obsessive rational analysis, grasping frantically for what can't be had, and embrace freedom as an agent navigating my circumstances.

With an innocent until proven guilty mindset, I transition my thinking. I choose to imagine every test confirming my wellness, not identifying recurrent disease. I no longer watch and wait, I live and observe.

∗   ∗   ∗

Having earned the privilege, I chomp at the bit to participate in a survivorship series at our wellness center. Virtually led group discussions include Pressure to Thrive, Managing Moods, Stress and Feeling Stuck, Survivorship Toolkits, Fear of Recurrence and Envisioning Your Future.

During the first class, I freeze during introductions. I will identify myself by my disease, or be the only one to opt out. I have been actively avoiding this defining moment. I would rather attend an Alcoholics Anonymous meeting and introduce myself there with a lie. As I turn my focus from inward to others, I know that I will choose the fair path. That I will meet other participants on a level playing field, with the diabolical truth. That we will connect, share, serve and receive one another in a safe and healing place.

∗   ∗   ∗

Wholly exposed and perpetually vulnerable, I am also dynamic, engaged, evolving and empowered. I know how to best serve myself, when to negotiate and when to perform, when to hold on and when to let go. In turbulent waters, I know when to float and when to swim. Instead of drowning myself fighting the tides, I ride the currents.

Lusting for life, I find myself again in countless little acts and magnified sensory experiences. Always and still detail-oriented, I relish the exquisite pleasure of micro-joys. Eating a perfectly ripe peach over the kitchen sink, the heady aroma captivates me as my teeth sink in to pierce the resistant velveteen skin and the sweet lush flesh, silky on my tongue, fills my mouth with nectar. I swallow pure bliss once more.

I find moments of satisfaction and pleasure, even in the isolation of my worst days, in the most deplorable circumstances and spaces. In the connectivity of my best days, I positively soar, resilient in body and mind. Passionately seizing my days with tenacity, I measure life not by what I have endured and evaded, but by every moment that I've spent living, independently and with extraordinary support.

*   *   *

From my greatest physical and emotional weakness, I will demonstrate my greatest strength. I will carry my burdens, navigate my terrain. Through grief, I know what I can bear.

In times of flux, I live with fear, not inside it. I refuse to cower, to pray, to beg. I stand up, I uncover my eyes. I mind my footing and then stand firm. I will kneel no more.

Inhaling deeply, I unfurl my spine, set my shoulders down and back, exhale, and raise my chin to the warmth of the sun. My hands drop to my side, and I breathe.

PHOENIX RISING

October 2020

"In order to rise from its own ashes, a phoenix first must burn."

Octavia Butler

A mythical golden bird associated with renewal and regeneration, the phoenix rises from the ashes of its previous life as a symbol of hope. Too deeply wounded to heal, yet determined to transform, that immortal bird lives inside my charred soul and flutters its torched wings.

I look back and see my ignorance, my fear, my weakness. Enlightened, I look in the mirror and see my strength, my power, my will. My efforts to rule my world cease when I focus on the present moment, using my inner voice to empower myself with calm and confidence in the now. I rest my body, nurture my mind and renew my resolve. Set down at a crossroads, I draw a new map.

*　　　　*　　　　*

I apologetically request copies of my hospitalization and surgical reports. In acts of gross perversion, I sift through thousands of pages of medical records, seeking and never finding answers and understanding in the unknown and unknowable. Following the torment of countless exhaustive attempts, I will never be able to reconcile the why.

Disease does not always cull the weakest of the herd, there may not be survival of the fittest. In our first world country, we live in a land of opportunity amid self-induced health crises. Nutrition and exercise are the most under-utilized preventative medication, as well as the most effective. Our rates of chronic disease in the masses are obscene, and we have diligently worked our way towards earning the highest global death rate for avoidable and treatable conditions.

In a society where the most miniscule discomfort evokes anxiety and its excuses, my threshold for petty trials and tribulations is low. I sin with wrath, internally condemning negligent people who so blatantly squander their wellness by electively abusing their bodies and minds. When the body is not revered as the temple that it is, I am judgmental and resentful, less virtuous.

*   *   *

In *The Great Battle of Fire and Light*, Tim Urban explores the battle between the primitive mind, experiencing life in survival mode, lack and competition, and the higher mind, experiencing life with presence, gratitude and compassion. While the wild and untrainable primitive mind drowns in negativity bias, the flexible, centered and open higher mind embraces personal evolution.

Ruled by semantics, I consider betrayal versus admiration, insecurity versus perseverance, recovery versus rebuilding, moving on versus moving forward. I think less about being deceived and how to recover trust, living in a body that was a liar, cheater and thief. I consider what I have endured, and bow to the body's innate ability to restore itself, without interference. My physical and emotional battle scars are reminders that I survived.

My experiences reveal my true capabilities and my powerhouse resources. Fear and strength will continue to reveal themselves layer by layer, and I can count on my spirit to take me wherever I need to go.

*   *   *

Now cultured in the field, I have learned a new language and found hope in the shadows of what is most likely a death sentence without a cure. Oncology terminology is carefully scripted to provide a sense of comfort in extreme duress. For the fortunately uninitiated, a *journey* with *infusions* might sound delightful. Best in this case not to call a spade a spade! This has been a brutal trek, a ruthless ordeal, a grueling and interminable haul.

Despite Nietzsche's popular 19th century claim, what doesn't kill you does not ipso facto make you stronger. Struggle doesn't automate resilience. The choice is ours, to roil in our turmoil or to roll up our sleeves in favor of the high road.

I use the prescribed jargon, however do not give up my vocabulary. My journey recall in the before is the bliss of hiking through unexplored rural regions of Italy, with only a Fiat 500 keeping our feet from the ground. My journeys in the after will be our adventures in Portugal and South America. Infusions will be fine organic tinctures that I sip from an old artisan mug, warming the palms of my hands. I will never define myself from the confines of a cancer setting or adopt a disease as my identity. I am so much more than the mass of my cells.

*   *   *

In *The Wisdom of Your Body: Finding Healing, Wholeness, and Connection through Embodied Living,* Hillary L. McBride, PhD explains the dominant influence of emotions on our sense of self and how central they are to our survival. The structure most deeply embedded in our brain hijacks the thinking brain in life threatening situations. Emotions have a purpose, yet we hush their innate wisdom. In a society that largely devalues the body and overvalues rational thought, discovering emotional controls at the helm of a crisis can be deeply disruptive. McBride encourages us to torch ideals that are restrictive, damaging and often unattainable. To improve our physical and mental health, we must be present and aware of our inner landscapes and treat ourselves with curiosity and kindness.

When we are hurting, what we need is patient understanding to prove to our whole brain-body system that we are safe, that whatever we went through is in the past, that it is not happening again in this moment. Generating this response internally will enable us to begin the process of healing from stress and trauma, even within moments after it occurs.

Both self-serving and accommodating by nature, I realize that compassion and mercy can and should be self-administered. I connect with what is right and wrong in my body and absolve myself of what I did and didn't do. Accepting and atoning with fortitude, shame ebbs and pride flows.

*   *   *

Though human lineage split from chimpanzee lineage around seven million years ago, and evil has always coursed through the veins of primitive and higher beings, progressive humanity has devolved in consideration, care and contact. I am disheartened by social and political perils and unrest, at home and globally. Our abused and neglected environment distresses me, and related toxins add to my multitude of paranoias. We pollute our bodies, homes and lands with products that pretend to improve our quality of life. Our material and consumable culture is deeply contaminated, from manufacturing, to use and consumption, to disposal. Everything man and machine made is subject to scrutiny. The depth and breadth of the situation is calamitous and overwhelming.

Despite all that, humanity has yet to go to hell in a handbasket in its entirety. I quell my panic by applying perspective and with more consciously considered choices. I cast down the devils and won't illuminate them with my overt attention. Instead, I honor and celebrate the angels, there are plenty to choose from. I set aside countless personal and general woes, refuse to surrender joy, and protect my spirit from the ills I cannot repair.

*   *   *

My elder stepdaughter marries her fiancée in an intimate ceremony that suits them both perfectly. With consideration and care, our small group braves gathering amid a pandemic to celebrate their life together. The bride and groom are genuine and loving. The bride's siblings are sensitive and protective, grounding touch posts of light in the dark shade of a beautiful day. My husband and I hold hands in unity, rejoicing in our enriched family.

We delay our return home for a short respite in the Smoky Mountains. During our post-wedding sojourn, we experience the ancient medical principle of vis medicatrix naturae, and the inherent healing powers of nature as we connect to the land, to our *terra firma*.

While some may live to conquer the Appalachian Trail, Camino de Santiago or Mount Everest, we explore a moderate foothill course and survey, collect and heal. Walking mountain roads, we descend and ascend over six hundred feet in elevation. From mortally injured, emaciated and collapsing, to walker, cane, brace and therapy dependent, to an inconceivable and victorious now.

*   *   *

Months later, my husband and I will travel to Iceland, where my aspirations guide my possibilities. I seek no medical counsel nor permission, I have already been told to live my life. I climb 370 steps, gripping the rail against 70 mph wind gusts, to reach the top of a waterfall on our first day. I mount an Icelandic horse, the only breed in the world that can perform five gaits, resulting in an allegedly more comfortable jaunt for the rider. My steed does not know how long it will take my body to heal from the wrack and ruin of surgery. Never carrying me into his fifth gear

127

flying pace, he rides rough and leaves me wholly shaken. Another equine encounter in a pasture ends with me gently pushing through the velvety muzzles of too many horses, circling me and vying for attention. A high-performance powerboat tour races us through the wild cold sea, delivering an adventure induced rush of adrenaline. Reckless and free, I drive too fast on the open roads and wait for my husband to tell me to slow down before I release my increasing pressure on the accelerator. I scale mountains and look down on valleys, awash in emotional reflections and realities. Perched on a boulder overlooking the vast, pristine landscape, I am utterly still, in a state of profound awe.

Despite pride being one of the seven deadly sins, I indulge euphorically and celebrate my toes touching new grounds. My appreciation and admiration for my beloved caregivers overshadows my sin. Without my good guides and gear, our collective wisdom and intellectual, technical and physical dedication, there would have been no advantages. These words would not exist, nor would I. The fibers of my being have been remade by my clinicians, family, friends, acquaintances, and even innocent strangers. Forever a part of me, my victories are shared.

*   *   *

Feverish and infatuated, I reinvented and dedicated my life to my husband with a vision. Now, while missing our innocence and physical liberties, I imagine nothing. I know his limitless depth of character intimately, there are no bounds to his devotion. I know what he is truly capable of, what we are truly capable of, how far we will go to stay together. Though we have now experienced extreme degrees of separation and solidarity, our relationship is ever fluid. Bruised and battered, we still lose track of where we each begin and end, even more so. There is so much beauty in the wreckage and as long as my heart beats, I will not let us go.

Decades ago, I read Nancy Milford's *Savage Beauty: The Life of Edna St. Vincent Millay* and fell a little bit in love with the feminist icon. A long-treasured passage from Millay's epic 1912 poem "Renascence" permeates me more now than ever before.

> *I know not how such things can be;*
> *I only know there came to me*
> *A fragrance such as never clings*
> *To aught save happy living things;*
> *A sound as of some joyous elf*
> *Singing sweet songs to please himself,*
> *And, through and over everything,*
> *A sense of glad awakening.*
> *The grass, a-tiptoe at my ear,*
> *Whispering to me I could hear;*
> *I felt the rain's cool finger-tips*
> *Brushed tenderly across my lips,*
> *Laid gently on my sealed sight,*
> *And all at once the heavy night*
> *Fell from my eyes and I could see,*
> *A drenched and dripping apple-tree,*
> *A last long line of silver rain,*
> *A sky grown clear and blue again.*
> *And as I looked a quickening gust*
> *Of wind blew up to me and thrust*
> *Into my face a miracle*
> *Of orchard-breath, and with the smell,*
> *I know not how such things can be!*
> *I breathed my soul back into me.*

*　　　　*　　　　*

After a spectacular display, the fall season draws to a close. When the trees release their leaves readying for winter, they remind me that I must let go to emerge anew.

There is less of me, there is more of me, I am transcendent…I am whole.   Fragile yet fierce, traumatized yet triumphant, insecure yet inspired, I dare to imagine the rest of my life.

THE AFTERMATH

"The season when to come, and when to go,
To sing, or cease to sing, we never know."

Alexander Pope

Though my wounds are no longer gaping, my grief still seeps. Filled with horror and wonder, in a state of lingering disbelief, I have mourned the life I thought I was going to have.

I have restored self-order, alive and mostly intact. My scars have faded and I have healed, but I do not recover because there is no going back to the before. Beneath a polished and carefully tended veneer lies the truth, I am a decimated, fragile version of my former self. My scriptures are solid in theory and spotty in execution. Tension vibrates beneath the surface of my skin. I hum in heightened awareness to a pervasive tick-tock and am unable to hush my active mind.

I know the hostilities and conflicts of war, as well as the peace that prevails. A cancer diagnosis has called me to the front lines of a battle, in a field littered with the bodies of those known and lost to the disease. Rarely is there one massacre, rather a series of small and large skirmishes, some consequential, others not. While death is seldom an imminent diagnostic outcome, the condition delivers an invitation to face mortality nonetheless. If we survive, we return with scars, identified by type and stage. Our bodies ravaged and our minds eternally altered in the after, no stone will be left unturned. Visible exteriors, hidden interiors, and psyches will all be inundated with shrapnel. We are sent back to the comforts of a home that will never feel the same, insecure in our surroundings. We return to relationships where we play different roles, adjusting with closeness or distance. Still tethered, with occasional temporary releases, we wonder when, not if, we will be called into combat again. We live within a calendar of mandated testing, both anticipating graduations and waiting to be dealt the fatal blow that awaits us.

*   *   *

Dates are etched into my subconscious and every November will launch a cycle of grief. I anticipate, counter and live with the Anniversary Effect's lashings, more acutely aware of the precious time I have left to live the best of my life.

I live in a house of cards, delicately balanced and rattled by the cancer connections that I continue to find in this rare yet related world. Now accustomed to being micromanaged by my well-known and trusted jailers, I am jolted and disoriented by change and influx. I am bewildered when roles shift or I am left to my own questionable devices. As much as I resisted being led, I still flounder in the freedom of release.

Stockholm syndrome dictates that I keep and protect my known resources. Scenes of my undoing and salvation are both distressing and comforting. With sentimental attachment to the hospital campus, cancer center and staff, I both despise and sickly yearn for their familiarity.

*   *   *

When my oncologist leaves the practice, I am devastated and take her abandonment personally. How can I live without her when she saved my life and guided me through the fires of hell with her able and gentle hands? I trust her implicitly, our bond is irreplaceable and I am leery of new practitioners.

Years after our last encounter, on a ship navigating South America and the Chilean Fjords, I will see an American Kestrel and think of her. An unusual visitor, unfortunately in decline, this land bird seeks respite onboard. North America's littlest falcon, while strikingly elegant, packs a predator's fierce intensity

132

into its small body, hunting by day and pouncing on its prey, seizing it with one or both talon-tipped feet. Courageous, the Kestrel does not hesitate to harass, attack or compete with larger creatures in its widespread territory. In stance, ferocity and power, my oncologist is admirably similar.

*   *   *

All of the aforementioned signs that I am at death's door still persist on a daily basis, thanks in part to the repercussions of surgery, chemotherapy, ongoing maintenance therapy, and possibly a yet to be discovered deadly condition.

Impressive tangents in which I expel frustration with a remarkably foul mouth point to Tourette's syndrome. In addition to lifelong perfectionism and obsessive-compulsive tendencies, I have become a prolific hypochondriac and now frequently exhibit classic symptoms of manic depression, multiple personality disorder and paranoid schizophrenia. Though clinically undocumented, I independently determine that these are all sure side effects of my disease and treatments.

I consciously release the tension in my permanently clenched jaw and slide my tongue over the wounds inside my unconsciously cannibalized cheeks. Intense flushing, vicious boiling over hot flashes and raging feverish night sweats disrupt my rest at all hours, my skin must be melting from my bones. Joint pain in my hands resolves with movement and a resurgence of synovial fluid, though should a sheet or limb inadvertently intercept my protected night claws, pain sears through my fingers and jolts me awake. My first steps are laborsome and belie my age by dozens of years. My pelvic floor is tight as a drum, my digestive system is a finicky miser and my bladder is a sensitive hyperactivist. Despite radiological evidence to the contrary, the chronic weight on my chest and dry cough must stem from a heavy heart, and I would swear that, at best, my inhibited breathing is due to a bale

133

of cotton bolls amassed in my lungs. From head to toe, random aches, pains and oddities sound alarm bells.

In genuine and well-acted macabre routines, I will die a thousand deaths over the course of my remaining days. It's not in my nature to stay put, and I cannot help swerving out of my lane to sidle up to medical professionals, though my diagnostic wisdom proves unreliable. I am still here, and the question of what and when remains.

*   *   *

As I still live and breathe, the professor will prove to be the sole practitioner with a crystal ball. The only person in my entire hemisphere to liken my future so blatantly to a poor statistical outcome, wholly discounting and underestimating my individuality and abilities.

He was not intentionally and exceptionally cruel, nor have others kindly protected me from a harsh truth. There is a time and a place for statistics, and my favored clinicians recognize the spirit behind the science, the exceptions to the rules.

With the benefit of time, I will concede to the professor and warm to destiny as a valid outcome. My life may take many different forms, the most critical of which I can neither predict nor control. *Que sera, sera…*

*   *   *

My past is about survival and controlling unbridled chaos. The minutes, hours, days, weeks, months and years following the before are the ones that redefine me, from victim to my own wilding warlord.

I share Sisyphus' scorn for the gods, hatred of death, and passion for life, though I hope to avoid his fate. After cheating death, Sisyphus is cursed and forever rolling a boulder up a hill in the

134

depths of Hades. Despite his eternal punishment, recollecting that he once held death in chains, he smiles. While he's pushing that rock, death has still not conquered him. The moral being, if the futility of a Sisyphean task with no preferable alternative is accepted without horror, we will be resilient and persevere in the face of adversity.

*   *   *

I follow my oncologist's advice and consider my legacy as a perspective informing my life. My core values and character, the total of my good and bad life experiences, and the footprints I will leave in my wake.

My journaling assignment has ended, no one is asking me to track my daily maladies and moods. My heart quickens when I realize that the journal can join all the other detritus, I no longer need it. Having one last look, I see beyond all the bad. There is so much good. It's the quotes that tug at my heartstrings. They are too inspiring to let go, and I begin to wonder. Are there people out there like me?

*   *   *

I read ovarian cancer memoirs written by pioneer women who were strong enough to survive and courageous enough to release their story, precious few exist. From brave amateur to the most sophisticated professional authors, all unique yet linked in mortal battle. Without exception, under the weight of dire circumstances, they all chose to empower themselves. Though faltering at times, there was a continuous current of strong will. An intent to survive, and to find and deliver positive purpose from their experiences. They heroically bared their bodies and souls, sharing intimate details of the most physically and emotionally challenging times of their lives. They generously offered comfort in kinship, gifting others with inspiration and hope.

I envision joining them, building an altruistic chronicle of my experience from the debris. I consider the value of my echo, in the quiet room of this secret society. Worthy or not, I commit to contribute to this remarkable sisterhood…to unfold my ovarian cancer journey.

In a cathartic act, I transcribe the most poignant passages in my journal into what will become *Living in Legacy* and relish liberating myself from those vile pages. Loathing and wanting to abolish the devil that had taken hold of me, I rip each sheet from its binding, knowing that I will never set eyes on the madness of my pencil markings again. Crumbling the pages into balls with furiously trembling hands, I loosen my grip and release my clenched fist to drop the smashed memories into the bin. Unshackled, my fingers are splayed wide open and I imagine the papers burning to ash. I destroy the journal in its entirety.

*   *   *

More than two years into a global pandemic that has now claimed millions of lives, with no sign of abating its virulent path, I regrettably let my guard down and contract COVID under social circumstances that I knew better to avoid. Still compromised and at high risk, my immune system suffers the intrusion and I am sick for the first time since treatment, and again frequently thereafter.

Just after I believe I have recovered, the exertions of travel and my social ambitions prove too much to bear and a severe rebound leaves me terribly ill and bedridden in a remote area of Italy. While I ponder death and endeavor to protect my extended family from my condition, my husband desperately wants to fly me home to receive known medical treatment and my parents stress over my incessant wracking cough. I refuse all requests to cease and desist. Malta bound on what may be our last expedition, I insist on making up for what we missed, knowing that I cannot yet bear the international return.

Subsequent CTs add to existing suspicious imaging, identifying worrisome changes in lymph nodes and ground-glass opacity in my lungs that will require follow-up and additional monitoring. All pressing concerns to add to my repertoire, along with growing studies regarding the short and long-term effects of the virus (cancer thrives in the nurturing environment of an inflammatory state). I loathe my poor judgment and my circle of trust again shrinks.

*   *   *

My new primary care physician takes the helm of my general health, closely monitoring my various conditions and complaints. In an ever more physically and emotionally distant world, he dares to express genuine concern and even warmly hugs me, bucking modern convention and who knows how many protocols. His sincere and compassionate care is as curative as any prescription that he could scribe.

Throughout our lifetimes, touch is a profound and critical human need. Babies can die from skin hunger and adults who are touched regularly live longer. Touch starvation robs the blood stream of the increased oxytocin garnered from sustained physical contact and increases feelings of stress, depression and anxiety. The pressure of a single fingertip has the power to lower blood pressure, improve moods and fortify immune systems.

Should every medical interaction that I have be an assault? Shame on our litigious society for harnessing the wholesome powers of integral healers!

*   *   *

When night falls and not a creature is stirring, I am very much alone and suffering. Still desperate to cling to a now I can't reach, I am unable to escape the imprint of trauma and am plagued with chronic secondary insomnia over the course of over a thousand nights. Living with the burdensome weight of being under constant threat, I do not feel safe enough to still my mind and cannot deeply relax. Starved for the oblivion of sleep, my rest is interrupted with migraines, hormonal fires, and runaway thoughts. I wake in dark early-morning witching hours, defenseless and regurgitating the horrors of what was and what may be, violently jousted between graphic flashbacks from my traumatic past and panicked visions of a terrifying future.

Lodged between a ruminating rock and catastrophizing hard place, I fail to exit the hamster wheel, to release my frenetic wandering imaginings, to calm myself with grounding exercises. Hyperaware of the related toll on my body and mind, I stress over triggering recurrence, over the loss of gray matter in my prefrontal cortex.

Exploring holistic eastern medicine practices, natural witchcraft and psychology, I am determined to read, work and will my way to wellness. Clearly modeling post-traumatic stress disorder and acute situational anxiety, I remain guarded and will spend over three years trying to Zen my way to peaceful sleep.

*   *   *

According to the troubled F. Scott Fitzgerald "In a real dark night of the soul, it is always three o'clock in the morning, day after day," but my highly adept physician will have none of that. I am finally gifted with the promise of peace when he steps into the fray to save me from myself.

During my first appointment, he identifies my neurologically inhibited stress response and long-depleted serotonin and devises a sensible treatment plan to address my body's chemical inability to achieve restorative sleep. My strength lies in acceptance, and I acquiesce to temporarily adding a low dosage selective serotonin reuptake inhibitor (SSRI) to my evening routine. Nearly giddy with relief, both exhausted and energized, I am determined to shed light on waves of oppressive darkness with that tiny tablet.

*   *   *

For two weeks, nightmares plague my chemically induced REM sleep, and I realize that I have had no dream recall during my longstanding insomniatic state. In the next month, unable to abandon my guard post, I easily fall asleep yet within minutes wake to a rush of panic and attempt to still my wildly beating heart with steadying deep breaths.

In the middle of the night, when I unconsciously fling my arm over my head in bed, I am instantaneously jarred from restless sleep and teleported to a CT table in the hospital. Shocked and alarmed, I immediately reposition. Less than one week later, I fling my arm over my head again and wake with the same reaction, though actively choose to relax. I reassure myself with the knowledge that I am in my bed, at home. Eventually, I am able to dismiss my memories to rest with both arms extended over my pillow. I am safe, and I am healing.

Ill spent nocturnal hours are whittled away, though I still can't shake my restless habits in their entirety. I am distraught by cognitive overload and would likely benefit from a lobotomy and/or electric shock therapy. After a few months of stable improvement, I quit the SSRI cold turkey.

*   *   *

Long after my scars have faded, a hammam attendant in Istanbul will ease me into subservience by telling me that I am her baby. She asks if I am hurt before scrubbing my body vigorously and enveloping me in billions of bubbles. Even the Ottoman Empire's ritual ablutions will not enable me to shed my skin. I am a marked woman.

Through intensive massage therapy, I learn that when physical trauma occurs, the muscles surrounding the injured area reflexively tighten to create stability. With emotional trauma, blunted disassociation spares the mind what it cannot bear. From a literal and figurative fetal position, a soft touch will release my defensive posture and be the antidote to the abuses I have endured, though the constant cacophony of my inner monologue drowns out the meditative music.

*   *   *

In 1817, Keats wrote about "negative capability"–being in uncertainties, mysteries, doubts, without any irritable reaching after fact and reason. Still suspicious, I cannot presume that all is well, yet I have learned to live with discord. I redefine my expectations and tentatively trust the future, despite being unable to justify my past.

Looking backward or forward with authority takes me away from the prize of the now. In a game of Tug of War, even when nothing matters more to me than beating the opposition, I mind my hands. When holding on is more painful than the relief of letting go, I release my grip.

Though not at peace, I have surrendered to my landscape. My only security is in knowing that I'm capable of dealing with whatever comes.

*   *   *

When I misassign meaning or significance with magical thinking, I remind myself of what is real versus perceived, that thoughts do not incite or protect. My inclination is to not plan beyond my next, and possibly last, supper. From being unwilling to frivolously invest in replacing a worn pair of shoes, I force the confidence to design a coded wedding anniversary ring. The centerpiece amethyst is powerful and protective, symbolizing peace and unification. It is my husband's birthstone. Paying tribute to him and securing our future for the next fifteen years, I indulge in a tentatively hopeful promise with all appendages tightly crossed. I hope to give him everything he has earned and deserves, and so much more than what my illness stole.

When a tiny diamond goes missing from my wedding band, instead of a false restoration, I opt to replace it with an emerald. The life-affirming stone symbolizes truth, love and hope. While it may not provide eternal life, as the Egyptians believed, the spark of green reminds me to embrace change with authenticity.

*   *   *

We celebrate my husband's birthday with a mixed media art acquisition, the piece is called *Have a Ball* by Gary Brown. Repurposed vintage papers include an illustration of a little blonde girl happily dropping a ball. The panel below her includes the following script:

DO YOU KNOW
why a Ball bounces?

When the size or shape of a body (whether solid, liquid or gaseous) is altered by the application of a force, there is a tendency for the body to return to its previous size or shape as soon as the force ceases to act. This tendency (which, of course, varies considerably in different substances) is known as elasticity. In the case of the hollow rubber ball bounced on a hard surface, both the rubber and the air inside are compressed to a considerable extent and being elastic cause the ball to bounce repeatedly. When it is bounced on a cushion, however, much of the force is expended in moving the cushion and consequently there is less compression of the rubber and air, and therefore less rebound.

*   *   *

Resembling the never quite satiated me of days long gone by, with reins now lax, I wildly forge ahead. To compensate my miserable year and possibly shortened life, I choose my obsessions wisely. I skirt being too still and enter my most prolific creative period. Manias of activity are tempered by rest, and I don't hesitate to opt out when I'm not inclined.

We boldly trade condo life for independence in a historic house and make it our home, finding solace in the property and grounds. The house and I share evident marks of a similar past. It survived a 1904 lightning strike when it failed to succumb to nature's forces and refused to burn to the ground. When we place the Greek flaming symbol of life at the entrance, I am grounded in humanity and hope. Protective evil eyes and haint blue porch ceilings ward off malevolent spirits. Woodland critters delight me, even the naughty bunnies. Light filtering through the old redbud tree and dancing sea oats settle my nerves. A roadside salvaged antique daybed is remade into a meditation bench, the griffon feet symbolize the union of the most powerful land and air animals in our great outdoors. Every act of preservation and investment is restorative, my paint- and dirt-stained hands heal with movement.

*   *   *

We celebrate our seventeen-year wedding anniversary in Norway. My prized and only souvenir is a collection of found fjord glass. From a ruined functional vessel, broken, no longer of value and long ago discarded, the ebb and flow of salty and sweet water eventually wear the fractured shards into velveteen softness. The more eroded, the more treasured. My feet are bare on the cold wet stones and I step into the shallow bank, seeking more. I spread my gems out and sort each piece by color, and then by feel. The pieces that are still working their way toward their best state are returned to the water's edge, for someone else to find. The pieces that I save will fringe a lampshade in our foyer, a moment of communion as we enter and exit the sanctity of our home.

*   *   *

Living in Legacy is alive, keeping me busy day and night, driving me mad. Unearthing and confronting my past, present and unknown future, I attempt to identify, make sense of and contain the unimaginable, to purge it all from my system. Every memory and reality tears into my delicately healing psyche, opening wounds I can scarcely accept having.

With much trepidation, I strive not to be shamefaced in attempting to share a portion of my broken heart. With unflinching honesty, in a deeply personal and raw narrative, I relinquish my last layer of protection. I delve into understanding the unthinkable to lay words to the unspeakable. From my greatest struggles to save my body, mind and soul, the moments that most viciously test my days and plague my nights, the benefit of hindsight, and the exceptional resources that have given me the vision and resolve to endeavor to survive.

I happen upon a tiny antique leather box in the shape of a book. Gold leaf lettering on its spine, *The Pleasures of Life*, is both a title and an encouraging sign. While more than the paltry sum I generally assign to my box fetish, it will be my inspiration, my compensation, my reward.

*   *   *

In *The Perfectionist's Guide to Losing Control: A Path to Peace and Power*, Katherine Morgan Schafler defines the fallacy of closure. Control, an ironically counterfeit non-sensible saboteur of power, fuels the desire for closure. On our own terms, we attempt to take a whole experience and reduce it down to one static piece, one story that doesn't change with a predominant theme and overarching sentiment. We streamline the remnant confusion in our internal world with logic and sense. We organize and catalog our pain, and choose which feelings to attach to which memories to exfoliate the rough surface of an experience to reveal a reassuringly pure and glistening core. Everything is clean and explainable, justified and righteous. We believe that closure has taken away our hurt. No longer penetrated by pain, we are officially done and our proverbial therapy paperwork is red-stamped HEALED!

As much as we would like to, we can't apply analytics to grief. Healing doesn't culminate in bullet-pointed certainty about anything, thoughts and feelings don't operate with an itinerary and we can cohabitate with happiness and difficult emotions.

According to Schafler, "Experiences swirl around in spheres. When you demarcate healing with midway points and finishing lines, you make healing a race and something that ends. Healing is neither. Spheres have no sides. Healing is less about establishing resolution and more about being able to center yourself in the parts of your life that remain unresolved. Some moments are devastating, retching, abominable, horrible. Period. We don't need to transmute every uncomfortable emotion into something shiny and useful. When you understand that closure is a fantasy, you have all the closure you'll ever need. People who heal are not the anointed ones who've figured out how to tie up all the loose ends; they're the ones who've pulled the string to something new."

*   *   *

The skies are dark with pregnant clouds and rain washes away half a century of sins on my fiftieth birthday. Though envisioning an intimate candlelit evening *al fresco*, I stay the course and adjust to the inclement weather patterns. During a brief cocktail hour reprieve, we walk the grounds and the blare of a tornado siren hastens our return to the safety of our longstanding structure. It may be an omen foretelling the year ahead, but I do not cry. I laugh happily. The blaze of fifty candles on our dining room table illuminates the faces of my loved ones, one of whom belts out spontaneous operatic odes. His magnificent voice carries from our ears to our souls, and out the open windows into the atmosphere. Second to South Africa, it is my favorite birthday ever.

*   *   *

Another mixed media art acquisition will serve as a guide in the second half of my life. Designed and fabricated by female artisans who have brazenly entered the male dominated field of metal work, the piece is called *The Wisdom of Words* by Things of Steel. Random steel letters are anchored with an *X*, *U*, and *W*. Reminders of where we are…at the core of our everything…enabled to choose our words to ourselves and others wisely.

As evolved creatures, perhaps our most unique characteristic is the depth and breadth of our language. I could easily spend the rest of my days pontificating, spewing disjointed, messy, horrifying, glorious thoughts on these pages. At what point are there ample words to capture the magnitude of events, at what point will I accept that it's time to stop rescripting, that this will never be a complete account, that my life isn't static and that I won't tempt fate with my last word? There is so much more, but this is enough.

It may be a perfect failure, but it is ready if not polished. My husband reminds me that there comes a point in every project where it's time to shoot the engineer and start production, that I am human and imperfect (more than recurrence and death, I fear a typo). On the eve of my four-year post-treatment milestone, the time has come to bring this magnum opus to a close. My story must be released to take flight, and I must land to rest.

*   *   *

A tiny museum in Nafplion, Greece houses a private collection of komboloi, the storied worry beads serve their owners as an amulet. A matchmaker guides me in selecting the strand that best suits me, as an aid for tranquility and meditation. It isn't the one made of olive pits, that fits securely enough in the palm of my hand to be smothered. It's the one made of fragrant nutmeg, that reminds me that there is no freedom in a clenched fist.

*   *   *

My feet are ice cold. Riddled with shame and paranoia, I fear that *Living in Legacy* is too personal to publish. That I will be exposed and vulnerable outside of my trusted clutch. That with too many sharp edges and an overabundance of sentiment, it is not fit for public consumption. That it will be offensive, discounted, and ill-received.

I love some of it, I hate most of it, and I deeply regret all of it. At the eleventh hour, I am too invested to turn back, to burn it all, to put it on a shelf. Torn between purpose and privacy, between courage and cowardice, I cannot have it both ways.

Because it was never for me, and I want nothing from it, I concede to the why... It is for my body and mind rescuing clinicians. It is for my soul restoring family, friends and acquaintances. It is for you.

*   *   *

Viktor Frankl's highly influential *Man's Search for Meaning* identifies the path towards spiritual survival. "Everything can be taken from a man but one thing: the last of the human freedoms— to choose one's attitude in any given set of circumstances. Between stimulus and response there is a space. In that space is our power to choose our response. In our response lies our growth and our freedom."

In a battle between integrity and despair, I choose integrity. Despair dictates that I reinforce the bars of my cell, and I refuse to be my own jailer. Though my body may be victimized and imprisoned by a disease, or not, it does not define me. To inform my mind, I choose a heroic heart and soul.

*   *   *

On the mountain roads and in the windswept valleys, I am a better navigator, a force of nature. Still a harrowing drive, it is one that is familiar. I know enough about the road behind and ahead of me to anticipate my journey, to release my white-knuckled grip, to accept the terrain. I know the hairpin turns and blind spots by heart, and study the map less. I strap myself in, grasp the wheel and drive towards life, immersed in my beautiful legacy.

*   *   *

The sound of The Beatles' "Blackbird" reverberates in my ear drums, though I crudely bang out my own version on the piano with a right-hand melody and left-hand march.

Waiting for this moment to arise, I see in the dead of night, I fly with broken wings. I am free.

REMARKABLE RESOURCES

"One life on this earth is all that we get, whether it is enough or not enough, and the obvious conclusion would seem to be that at the very least we are fools if we do not live it as fully and bravely and beautifully as we can."

Frederick Beuchner

BOOKS

Being Mortal: Medicine and What Matters in the End, Atul Gawande

Maybe You Should Talk to Someone: A Therapist, Her Therapist, and Our Lives Revealed, Lori Gottlieb

Memoir of a Debulked Woman: Enduring Ovarian Cancer, Susan Gubar

Pretty Sick: The Beauty Guide for Women with Cancer, Caitlin M. Kiernan

The Body Keeps the Score: Brain, Mind and Body in the Healing of Trauma, Bessel Van Der Kolk, M.D.

The Perfectionist's Guide to Losing Control: A Path to Peace and Power, Katherine Morgan Schafler

The Ultimate Guide to Ovarian Cancer: Everything You Need to Know About Diagnosis, Treatment, and Research, Benedict B. Benigno, M.D.

The Unseen Body: A Doctor's Journey Through the Hidden Wonders of Human Anatomy, Jonathan Reisman, M.D.

The Wisdom of Your Body: Finding Healing, Wholeness, and Connection through Embodied Living, Hillary L. McBride, PhD

DOCUMENTARIES

Rising Strong: Manifesto of the Brave and Brokenhearted, Brené Brown

RSA Short: Blame, Brené Brown

RSA Short: Empathy, Brené Brown

TED Talk: The Power of Vulnerability, Brené Brown

TED Talk: What Almost Dying Taught Me About Living, Suleika Jaouad

TED Talk: Yes, I survived cancer. But that doesn't define me., Debra Jarvis

PHILOSOPHIES

In *Happiness Becomes You*, Tina Turner presents highlights in each of Buddhism's ten worlds.

1. HELL
    Positive: Personal experiences of deep suffering can lead us to the desire to help others find their way out of their own suffering.
    Negative: Hopeless despair; the inability to see oneself and others clearly; self-destructive tendencies.

2. HUNGER
    Positive: Aiming to achieve goals; yearning to have more.
    Negative: Greed; hedonism; insatiable desires.

3. ANIMALITY
    Positive: Healthy instincts to survive and to protect and nurture life.
    Negative: Acting only from instinct; threatening the weak

and fearing the strong.

4. ANGER
   Positive: Righteous passion to fight injustice; creative force for change.
   Negative: Egotistic self-righteousness; destructive competitiveness; conflict.

5. TRANQUILITY
   Positive: Neutral state of peacefulness; ability to act with humane reason.
   Negative: State of passive inactivity; unwillingness to tackle problems; laziness.

6. HEAVEN
   Positive: Sense of pleasure and happiness; heightened awareness; feelings of appreciation for being alive.
   Negative: Short-lived elation that is typically self-oriented; wish for fleeting gratification to repeat can lead to excess.

7. LEARNING
   Positive: Striving for self-improvement by studying new concepts through others' teachings.
   Negative: Tendency to become self-centered; dismissive attitude towards others with less experience or knowledge.

8. REALIZATION
   Positive: Gaining wisdom and insight through one's own learning and personal observation of the world.
   Negative: Lacking a broad view of life due to self-absorption; feelings of superiority over others.

9. BODHISATTVA
   Positive: Compassion; acting selflessly for others without expectation of reward.

Negative: Neglecting one's own life; feeling contempt for those one tries to help.

10. BUDDHAHOOD
Boundless wisdom, courage, and compassion; a grand life force that illuminates the positive aspects of each of the other nine worlds. Buddhahood is the only life condition that has no negative aspects.

REPORTS & RESEARCH

All of Us Research Program, National Institutes of Health

American Cancer Society

Count Me In

National Ovarian Cancer Coalition (NOCC)

Ovarian Cancer Research Alliance (OCRA)

CALL TO ACTION

Ovarian cancer is the deadliest cancer in its class and affects women of all ages, without discrimination. More than 80% of affected women are diagnosed at an advanced stage because early-stage disease is usually asymptomatic and symptoms of late-stage disease are non-specific. This rare disease is too common and diagnoses and deaths are alarmingly on the rise, globally.

Learn more at ocrahope.org.

AUTHOR'S NOTE

While the physicality of ovarian cancer serves as the catalyst for informing this memoir, the countless borrowed and found inspirational perspectives are not confined to a class of disease. For whatever reason a wayward soul may hunger to re-know itself, though individual experiences reign unique, I believe we all share a base desire to find comfort in pain and hope in despair. Should these pages serve to enlighten or inspire others, in body or spirit, they will have been well worth scripting.

*   *   *

I am the sum of everything and everyone in my life. The dear family and friends that read my drafts provided me with questions and answers that enabled me to better hone my voice, I am profoundly appreciative.

*   *   *

When I changed the course of my life, notes to my husband captured the depth of my adoration, yet everything in our before pales in comparison to the wisdom of our now. This book is my greatest love letter, and only begins to express what makes my heart beat and soul take flight.

We generally don't exchange presents, but his most generous gift to me was a found newspaper cutting. Saint Teresa of Calcutta's scripture captures the whole of what life is, and the path to a meaningful legacy…from our first breath to our last.

Life is beauty, admire it. Life is a dream, realize it. Life is a challenge, meet it. Life is a duty, complete it. Life is a game, play it. Life is a promise, fulfill it. Life is sorrow, overcome it. Life is a song, sing it. Life is a struggle, accept it. Life is a tragedy, confront it. Life is an adventure, dare it. Life is luck, make it. Life is precious, do not destroy it. Life is life, fight for it.